WRITTEN BY BEN COOMBER

HOW TO BE AN AWESOME PERSONAL TRAINER

Inspire greater change in your clients, have a better work-life balance, get better results, achieve greater job satisfaction and become a more successful trainer.

Self-Published by Ben Coomber Ltd

First Edition, Dec 2016

Copyright 2016

ISBN: 978-0-9956783-0-9

Book designed by Seven Seven Creative Solutions

Book edited by Jane Black

This book has been inspired by the beautiful industry we work in, fitness, and the
dream I have for its continual positive evolution.

Who is Ben Coomber?

Why do people always write this part of their book in the 3rd person. Did someone else write it for them?

This is my book, let's play by my rules...

My name is Ben Coomber. I'm a coach, speaker, educator, and pursuant of an AWESOME life. I'm always striving to be better in everything I do.

I first got into the fitness industry after a battle with obesity, IBS, ADHD and other classic issues: low self-esteem, lack of confidence and awareness of who I truly was.

Getting fit allowed me to build my identity and truly define the person I knew I could be. I then went on a journey to become a personal trainer, nutritionist and massage therapist and at the time of writing this book, I've developed my work and business into public speaking, teaching and coaching online. I aspire to benefit both the personal trainers of this world and the everyday folks just trying to be a little more AWESOME each day.

I'm the owner of The BTN Academy, an online nutrition and fitness education company and I also own and run Awesome Supplements, an ethical research-based nutrition supplement company.

I travel the world speaking, teaching and sharing my thoughts on all aspects of fitness, nutrition, diet, health, lifestyle, personal development, business and being AWESOME.

For the personal trainers of this world, this book is for you. I really hope it inspires you to create a positive impact on the fitness industry...

Other ways to find me and what I do:

Ben Coomber Radio – My #1 rated health and fitness podcast, available on iTunes and other podcasting apps and media players

All over social media – Facebook, Instagram, YouTube, my website - if all this social media stuff is still around by the time you read this book!

My website: www.bencoomber.com

The BTN Academy – For when you decide to take your nutrition education to the next level, we're here for you: btn.academy

Awesome Supplements – If you want to use an ethical supplement brand that's research proven and honest in everything that it does, while simplifying and innovating in the world of supplementation: www.awesomesupplements.co.uk

Other books I have written to date available at www.bencoomber.com:

The Nutrition Blueprint

The Sports Nutrition Blueprint

A Beginners Guide To Lifting Weights

An Intermediates Guide To Lifting Weights

Nutrition For Kids

As well as many other short books, e-books and other beneficial musings online, have a hunt around and I promise you'll find lots of good stuff!

Dedication

To all the personal trainers that choose to be AWESOME at what they do

Here's to you.

Contents

INTRODUCTION

I used to be a BAD personal trainer.

I had all the knowledge in the world but something was missing. If anything, thinking I knew it all was worse than if I knew nothing at all. Back then, I wish I'd equipped myself with the skills I'm going to discuss with you in this book. You see, being a world class personal trainer and getting clients their best results, cultivating a thriving business and achieving genuine job satisfaction requires far more than knowledge alone.

I've spent years learning and refining my craft, forever acquiring more knowledge in the hope that I would get the best results any trainer could ever achieve. Course after course, you name it, I've studied it: body composition, health and disease, systems biology, chemistry, nutritional supplements, movement coaching, strength and conditioning, massage therapy. The list goes on.

Yet somehow my results felt mediocre. I wasn't happy achieving mediocre results in only 30-40% of my clients at the best of times. I also didn't have a thriving business. My business was OK, but I'm not one for settling for OK and neither should you. In the early days I decided to be a personal trainer for two reasons: to inspire and share the life changing journey that got me into health and fitness, and to have the flexibility, enjoyment and all the benefits of owning your own successful business, the life of being self-employed. It's the dream right?

At this point in time I was doing neither successfully. Something had to change.

It wasn't until I started to master the art of business; appreciating the skill of psychology, delivering amazing customer service, understanding consumer dynamics, developing marketing skills and applying the principles of time management and mindset into my daily routine that my personal training business really took off.

Anyone can read books and gain knowledge, but that's not what makes a great coach. It's one of the things I dislike about the fitness industry: we operate in a practical world yet so many people are consumed with taking more theory based courses, reading even more books and adding yet another certificate to their name without really understanding the knowledge that has been acquired.

To become the best requires practical hands on work: taking the time to work with client's day to day, trialling ideas in a practical setting and taking tests that challenge you on a case study basis, not just multiple choice tests that force you to recall a fact. In other words, learning by doing, feeling, engaging, conversing, and being challenged by real world examples of the problems we all face with our clients.

If you are considering courses for your future development, which you should as we're in an industry that is always evolving, ensure you are taking courses that challenge you with the test, that do seem hard, being a great coach doesn't come from easy courses or multiple choice tests.

There is no point in having the certificate on your CV if it hasn't improved what you do as a coach, that's just for appearance sake, and that helps no one.

I expect a lot from myself. I want the best and I want to be the best I possibly can be and so should you. Every day should be a pursuit to better yourself as a person, as a practitioner and as a master of your trade. This is where real satisfaction comes from in life: mastering what it is you want to do, living and breathing your passion and being pretty damn good at it too.

Don't expect any short cuts from this book.

Sure, I'm going to teach you the skills that promise to make you an incredible coach. But you need to commit and put in the work. Hard work is severely underrated in any environment; you want to be great at something, you must put in the work.

You want to sculpt your ultimate physique? Work hard consistently in the gym.

You want to be rich? Commit to your business or your job and invest wisely.

You want to learn to master your mind? Take part in daily meditation practice.

You want to be as healthy as humanly possible? Eat lots of fresh real food daily

If you want to have a successful personal training business, put the work in and hustle on the gym floor or out in your community. Don't shy away behind a few

Facebook posts and cross your fingers in the hope it'll bring you clients. No amount of success comes from skipping the hard work; everyone that is successful, unless they come up with something truly unique (only 0.1% of people), have put in the work.

People ask how I became successful. The answer: I put in the work.

From aged 22 to 26 I dedicated my life to my business and worked on my trade as a coach: applying, failing, listening, understanding, learning, and progressing. From age 26 to the present day I'm still working my backside off.

In building my vision I still fail; I still learn from my mistakes and I'm still progressing and working on being the best coach that I can be. The difference now is that I can do this in a more structured, educated and assured way. At least I hope so.

Failure teaches you great things: it refines you and gives you the ability to be more successful. No one starts by knowing it all, far from it. Everyone has failed on the path to greatness so be willing to fail. I was and I still am. It's something that makes me great.

As your career grows you'll find the risks get bigger, the numbers grow larger and often there is more at stake. But experience teaches you to be more prepared for the outcomes. Often our failed experiences guide us into managing a situation and predicting the best outcome for us to take.

Don't think that the route to becoming an awesome personal trainer is an easy one. There is guaranteed hard work ahead. But hard work doesn't have to mean ten years of misery on the horizon. You have the ability to choose the actions on your path.

It all comes down to you: your personal dreams, wants and ambitions. Where do you honestly want to be as a coach? What does being an awesome personal trainer look like to you?

Only you can answer that by being truly honest with yourself. How many hours do you want to work? How many clients do you want to train? What type of clients do you want? What does your life look like when you 'make it'?

Mapping these ideas out creates vision and this is the foundation of your career plan. Without vision there is no real plan.

If you're reading this you might be a coach or personal trainer looking to improve your business: perhaps you want to achieve greater results for your clients - maybe you want to attract more clients, charge a higher rate for your services, create greater job satisfaction or build a better work life balance within your own gym or at a gym you work in. If any of those topics are the reason for you picking up this book, they're all perfectly good reasons to do so. But we need to shape your vision and be a lot clearer on how all of this looks and feels in order to bring your ideas to life.

Remember, vision is the foundation of your plan that you will form from the guidelines in this book. Be clear on your vision.

Let's say you have 10 clients training with you 1-2 times a week, generating you 15-18 hours of quality personal training sessions each week. Let's say you want to increase your sessions to 30 hours consistently each week while creating an improved work life balance, to work less unsociable hours, all while developing a more streamlined business model.

I'm going to teach you that and more. Implement what I teach you in this book and your goals, dreams and your vision could be achievable in a matter of months, if not weeks, if you commit to putting in the work (and doing the 'lock in').

Everyone is different and it might take longer than that, but if you commit to the work you can have a thriving personal training business or gym within 3-6 months if you sit down, plan, and follow the topics I talk about in this book.

For now let's get you to where you want to be. Let's get your business thriving, get you happy, get you less stressed, get your business organised, and be an AWESOME personal trainer. Let me help you achieve the dream you set out for yourself the day you decided to become a personal trainer.

But before we start (I know, you are motivated and pumped to get going and just implement the techniques in this book, but we need some context to lay a foundation), let me share my story with you and where this all began...

My story and how I realised I was a BAD personal trainer

It took me quite some time to realise that I wasn't the best personal trainer in the world.

I lost 5 and a half stone when I was 18 and was inspired to become a personal trainer through my own battle with obesity and several other health issues I had at the time. My transformation was so life changing that it ultimately changed my career choice. I left a career destined for acting to pursue personal training to teach others about the power of nutrition and movement.

(If you would like a lot more context and information on my transformation and weight loss journey, as well as lots of free learning, hit up my website www.bencoomber.com and look in the interviews area of my shop. All my past interviews are stored there where others have probed on my journey and my learnings from multiple angles).

After my transformation, I invested in my education. I learned a lot of cool stuff which lead me to become a nutritionist, personal trainer and massage therapist and I was fortunate enough to have some money put aside to do these courses, studying a great deal in a relatively short space of time. At this stage in my life, I studied mostly through the CHEK Institute and immersed myself in as many aspects of health and movement coaching that were available to me at the time.

So much knowledge I had acquired...

I felt bulletproof. In my mind I had all the skills to become the best personal trainer in the world.

But, in short, I became arrogant. I felt I knew it all; all I needed now was for people to listen, apply the knowledge I'd be giving them and success would be theirs.

I coached for 9 months in a private facility as a self-employed personal trainer before I got itchy feet and at aged 21 went to university. There I continued to coach in a Fitness First gym; my first experience of a commercial gym environment.

But before we get ahead of ourselves, let's address why I left my first gym, 'ReFresh Fitness' in Ipswich. At the time, I thought I was too good for the place; I assumed that the people there, my fellow coaches Ben and Jo who owned the gym, couldn't teach me anything more and the only way I could get any better was to be in an environment that allowed me to continue learning. At that point in time I had an insatiable appetite for learning as much as humanly possible and the next logical step was to attend university.

Was I legitimately not learning in my current environment, or was I trying to learn the wrong stuff? Or maybe I was not aware of the right assets I needed to learn and what Ben and Jo could teach me?

Some of my reasons for leaving the gym for university were legitimate, and some were not. Being younger and more immature at the time, I felt I had taken on too many adult responsibilities and if I'm being honest, I wasn't ready for it. I didn't feel like an adult; I wanted to live it up a bit more before work got a bit too serious. If I were to develop and improve my intrapersonal skills then I needed to be in an environment where I felt safer, less intimidated by the pressure and freer to develop at a pace I was happy with.

And so it was, I decided to go to university to study Sports Science, eventually bagging a place at Hull University on their Sports Coaching and Performance course. Within two weeks I was on my way and living the dream!

Self-awareness

One of the first steps in any journey of personal mastery is self-awareness, so please take note; if there is a single lesson you take from this book, let it be this. To be fully aware of your thoughts, emotions, assets, character traits and all the things that make you 'you'. It's an essential part of the self-improvement process.

(Fact is, you will get lots of lessons from this book, if you are open and ready for them, so please don't rush, and be ready and receptive to ideas and change).

At 18 I knew I was unhealthy, fat and unhappy.

Self-awareness allowed me to change that situation. And at this turning point in my life and career, I was becoming self-aware of the choices I was making. I wanted to be in an environment where I could have fun and would be able to bridge the gaps in my knowledge of biology, anatomy, physiology, psychology and biomechanics. That was one of the key reasons for choosing a degree in Sports Science. But there were other, more unsavoury reasons for my choice to leave. Deep down I felt better than the environment I was in and while I'd never vocalise that to others, it was an honest emotion. But it was an emotion that would become apparent in my work; I was an arrogant personal trainer and I didn't truly care or understand my clients, I thought I was above them, that I held the power and that people should just listen.

In hindsight, my reasons for going to university were all correct and justified at the time. If I hadn't have left I don't think I would be the person I am today. What happened next, a true turning point in my journey, would never have happened. So yes, things do happen for a reason, and we could argue that I could have learnt a lot from my current environment at ReFresh Fitness with Ben and Jo, if I had been open and receptive to it, but that obviously wasn't my life path. These were just the steps it took for my life path to open up in front of me.

It was at university (I'm now 21), in a Fitness First gym in Hull, that I realised I was a bad personal trainer. During my first 18 months working here I was more of a regurgitator than a personal trainer. I could tell everyone what to eat, why to eat it, how to eat it, how to move, why to move and could write some seriously funky training and diet plans. I knew how to impress (well, I thought so) my clients.

But I only managed to get results in around 30-40% of my clients, at best.

Why won't clients follow my amazing advice? Are they stupid? Are they not ready to change? Do they not want it badly enough? Do they like cake too much?

It was none of the above, it was me. I was the problem. I didn't take the time to appreciate and understand my clients as human beings.

How did I realise this?

The gym had a balcony section of free-weights, an area where you could stand and look down onto the busiest part of the gym. Quite often I would stand on the balcony observing the gym to see what people were doing, but also to parade my peacock chest and be noticed like an elite trainer like me, should do.

'Look at me, I'm the best'. Literally.

It was at my watch post that I was taught my very first lesson as a personal trainer. It was here that I witnessed the art of being a good human being and one of the key fundamentals of being a good personal trainer.

Each day I'd observe the gym's most popular personal trainer, racking my brains from afar: "How the hell does this guy have a waiting list for clients? He's a knuckle head!". The trainer in question was Tom Cowen, Fitness First Hull's most popular trainer. At first I put his success down to his appearance; if I was female I'd probably want to be trained by him. Yeah, he was a good-looking lad, that's why.

But it was nothing to do with his looks, it was what he did that mattered.

Day after day I would watch Tom train his clients. They would come in, jump on a piece of cardio equipment while he stood and talked to them for a good 10-20 minutes depending on the client before any of the 'real work' began.

"What client in their right mind pays someone to stand next to them and chat while they warm up on a piece of cardio equipment?" was my thought at the time. What a waste. Surely they could do that in their own time?

I couldn't work it out. What was it about Tom that made him the most popular trainer in the gym? He was always busy, yet here I was struggling along, never having any more that 2 or 3 clients at a time and I had the most advanced kick as programs in the gym.

Perhaps I was over qualified for this place? Perhaps people couldn't handle my knowledge? Perhaps they weren't ready....

Then I started to see what he did, and it was simple: he genuinely cared about his clients.

Now it wasn't that I didn't care for people; I thought I cared, but in hindsight I was caring about the wrong things. As a trainer I was always looking beyond the client to the things that, in my head, were most important for their success: the system, the diet, the exercise and the movements we were covering in the session. I was so excited to get my knowledge out there and prove to the client, and to myself, that I held the key to the things they needed to better their bodies. I never stopped to take note of their REAL needs.

Tom and I took two distinctly different approaches. When I got a client in I assessed them, outlined a plan, talked them through all their diet, training needs, movement and lifestyle choices and wrote them a new way to live. Everything all at once.

What did Tom do? He listened. It was that simple.

He took time to truly understand his clients: their wants, their needs, their problems, what makes them tick, what they valued, what they enjoyed, what they hated and their real reasons for being in the gym. And more.

Tom spent so long understanding the true nature of his clients that when it was time for them to implement his advice, it was often carried out with ease.

Those 10-20 minutes Tom spent talking to his clients while they warmed up on the treadmill were the most valuable part of the session, for both the client and for Tom. They would literally just chat: understanding one another, sharing stories, wants, desires and problems. They chatted about trash they had watched on TV, things that happened at work, general gossip and then finally the reasons they were in the gym in the first place and what they were going to achieve together.

People rarely buy knowledge. People buy off people.

Think about your own experiences here. If you've ever bought knowledge it's often because a level of trust or respect has been built up in some way beforehand, before any money has been exchanged.

You might have bought this book because you respect my work and what I do. While we may never have spoken together in person, I have done enough to make you trust and respect my work enough for a simple transaction of knowledge to have taken place; you have traded your money in exchange for my knowledge that you can go away and apply.

For me, this was the best baptism of fire I could receive. I now understood the missing link in becoming a great personal trainer, I had to care. I had to take the time to understand people if I was going to succeed in my business, I had to appreciate their wants, desires, motives and drives. So I started to spend time learning and observing some more.

Only when you are truly self-aware can you progress. It's so important to recognise this.

Please don't fear the thought of change. There might be things that you don't like about yourself for now and that's alright. This is the first step in the process of bettering yourself: identifying aspects of your character you can improve on, then putting strategies in place without them negatively affecting what you do and how you behave.

I knew that psychology and mind-set varied amongst different people but at the time I wasn't naturally good at understanding what it was that made people tick. I didn't consider others to be as good as I was, I was the best. This was partly a lack of development and skill on my part and lack of awareness of others, but also partly down to immaturity. If I didn't have the skills to take me to the next level, then I needed to learn them. If I wanted to be an AWESOME coach, I had to be more Tom Cowan.

There are 2 ways that you can learn to be a practitioner of your trade:

1. Watch, listen, observe, understand, experiment and explore.
2. Actively learning through reading, watching videos and taking part in courses.

Both are fundamental; you can't have one without the other. Education gives you the information and the understanding to be able to quantify and guide your coaching processes, whilst giving you a grounding for any assumptions you have on any given topic. On the other hand, the skill of being present, observing, being critical and listening are important for contextualising and applying what you've learned to the real world, to real people.

I started by doing just that. And looking back, this is probably the skill I am most grateful for. Learning by observing Tom working with his clients and quietly watching the world go by would be one of the best skills I could master. If I could understand people, what makes people tick, the problems they have, situations they can't solve, and the reasons they do things, then I could help them. Both as a trainer and as a business owner.

And to this day this is where most of my education largely comes from: observing the world, being present, and understanding what people do and why they do it. You can read as many books as you want and take as many courses as possible, but unless you are present in a situation and know how to apply your knowledge to people and to problems, it's all useless information.

That is why I've been so outspoken towards fitness industry courses that are based on reading a book and taking a test to get a certificate. It doesn't create a good personal trainer, at least not in 95% of cases. Not many people learn effectively from this style of teaching and often don't have the practical awareness to implement the knowledge from theory alone. Often, true knowledge acquisition comes from guided, interactive and visual learning.

I now have a good understanding of people, problems and the coaching environment. If I read a research paper, I know when and how to apply this knowledge in a practical setting. Yet there are a lot of coaches who struggle to contextualise this information in the real world with clients. We need courses that are practical, hands on, engaging and interactive, because that's the reality of the real world.

I used to treat my clients like a book or a set of circumstances. When I assessed my clients, worked out what they needed and expected them to apply it and get results, I only had a 20-30% success rate, 40% at best. Why? I simply wasn't understanding all the dynamics at play: the wants, desires, emotions, needs, and the problems people had. And that was the process I had to change.

I believe theory only gets you so far when you work with a real person.

So I now decided to spend my time on the gym floor helping people, talking to them, building rapport, advising, and creating connections. At that point in time I didn't know Tom all that well. He was always busy training clients then clocking off down to Prinney Ave (the trendy drinking hotspot in Hull at the time). But even in the brief moments of speaking to Tom I felt like he cared about me. He would say hello, ask how I was and put his hand on my shoulder as we shook hands. When talking to me he'd look me in the eye and seemed genuinely interested in my responses. He would always reply with a focus on me, it was never about him even if our encounter was 10 seconds long, I felt valued; nothing was arbitrary or fake.

This was a key lesson for me. It wasn't about being on a treadmill per se with a client for 15 minutes chatting trash before we started the session, although by all means do that for some of the early session you have with a client if you feel it is appropriate. It was about spending time learning about them as a person and finding that level of where to start them off. However you build this into your practice as a coach, ensure there are periods of time in the early days where you get plenty of time to talk, bond, and understand one another, that you genuinely get a chance to engage in their needs and emotional state.

Interactions like this made me realise there was another aspect of my character that I had to change: I was far too judgmental. Being judgmental is often a natural thing we humans do to protect ourselves from people and situations we are unsure about. In judging others we can see their flaws and in some ways, it makes us feel a little better about our own insecurities. It makes us feel superior.

But in the world of personal training you cannot judge anyone until you know the person or the situation.

To put my judgemental self into context and prove a point, we need to fast forward to a few years later. I remember a situation when I was working back home in Ipswich at a David Lloyd gym and applying my new found skills, trying my best to turn my business into a success (I got fully booked in 5 weeks from applying what I had learned; compare that to only 3-4 clients after 5 months in that Fitness First gym in Hull). But more on that later.

(You'll have to excuse this book jumping around a little with my story, but it's the best way I can convey it, and also the lessons within it. Keep up, you'll be fine).

So, I saw a guy sitting on a chest press machine pumping out reps. He was working hard but his technique was painful and I knew I should step in and help him before he seriously injured himself. Before I stepped into the situation, I automatically judged him as I shaped him up as potential client material (every person is a potential client after all).

As I approached him, my mind was full of thoughts:

"What's the point in even speaking to this guy, he won't ever be a client"

"He's too young, he won't have enough money"

"He won't understand the benefits of personal training"

"He's just here to lift weights with his mates, I probably shouldn't even say anything"

"He probably won't listen to me, he looks arrogant"

We can all find an excuse to avoid talking to someone and I was doing a great job convincing myself that he wasn't worth the effort. But I had a word with myself, put all my judgements aside and decided to give this guy some advice on his technique.

As it turns out, he really appreciated the advice. He had struggled with a pain in his shoulder during his chest sessions and the improvements to his technique immediately alleviated the pressure on his anterior deltoid.

I left him to carry on with his session. Ten minutes later I helped him with another exercise. "What's your name?" he asks.

"Ben"

"You're a PT right?"

"I am, yeah"

"Ah awesome. I like what you do. I've seen a few of the PTs in the gym and thought about getting some sessions. I know I could be training better and I want to make progress, but all the PT's seem arrogant so I haven't bothered asking".

It was at this point I was slapping myself for judging this guy, how could I be so stupid!

I then asked, "What is it that you do?"

"I work in sales," he replied, "And I'm f**cking good at what I do. So before you ask, yes I can afford personal training, so how about you start training me. I'm up for doing 3-4 days a week".

I held my head in shame.

Here I was thinking this young guy was probably arrogant, didn't have enough money to train with me and probably wouldn't appreciate the help of a personal trainer. Instead, it turns out he earned a good wage, was motivated to train, wanted to train multiple times a week and was a genuinely decent human being.

Why did he choose me?

We could put it down being in the right place at the right time, but isn't that just life? If the truth be told, some people appear to be lucky because they do the work required to succeed; they put in the effort and by doing more and showing up consistently, their efforts pay off.

Being on the gym floor, marketing your business and getting more clients is a numbers game. If you speak to 20 people you might strike up 10 positive conversations. Out of those 10 conversations, 5 lead to a more in-depth chat. As you get talking, 3 of those chats will have you utilising your advice giving out meaningful information on a workout or a situation. Eventually out of those 3 people, 1 signs up as a client. The more people you talk to and build rapport with, the greater the connections you make. The output results in more clients and a more successful business.

Now before we continue, I feel we need a brief re-cap. I don't want you to miss any lessons I feel are key, so, what should you be mindful of at this stage?

1. Self-awareness is key. Become self-aware and truly master your destiny

2. Understand people and spend time creating connections

3. Never judge a potential client. Don't pass judgement until you take the time to get to know the person

If you applied those 3 key lessons today I guarantee you will become a far more successful trainer and a better person. In fact, I might stop writing now; whatever you paid for this book has already been repaid.

I mean what I say. Apply those 3 simple ideas and so many good things will happen in your life. But only if you go through the process and put in the work.

Now as a side note I want to mention how I want you to read this book. I don't want you to sit down one Sunday afternoon and smash through every chapter in one sitting. Don't expect to learn and apply everything you read all at once, it's just too much.

We need to slowly build habits and change how we do things over time; give each process the necessary time needed to apply what you've learned. This will also ensure you avoid skipping any fundamental ideas that could benefit your career. It might be a good idea to read one chapter a week, then spend time planning ways to implement the ideas.

We learn too passively these days, listening to podcasts, watching videos and moving on to the next best thing without fully appreciating and reflecting on what we have learned, and thus never truly implementing the work.

Read, reflect, apply, and put in the work. And continue to refine and improve over time.

Anyway, enough side notes. Let's fast forward to the present day. I've been a personal trainer, I've been a coach, I've been a massage therapist and now I've transferred those skills to a bigger stage, using my brand of public speaking to educate others on becoming great personal trainers in their own right. I've applied the same skills from this book to my role as a public speaker, writer and educator; the only difference is that I'm doing it on a bigger scale.

So here we go. Let's dive into this book as I teach you how to be an AWESOME personal trainer through my journey from personal trainer to public speaker, business owner and leader to others.

P.S. Learn, reflect and apply.

P.P.S. Be self-aware, always.

CHAPTER 1
LET'S TALK ABOUT YOU

This book opened with my story and how I started to turn it around from being a bad personal trainer to the coach I am today. Now it's time to talk about you. Let's start with some considerations for your personal actions around your clients and how you present yourself within your environment.

Now remember the introduction and my PPS: be self-aware, always.

This is absolutely fundamental to this chapter as I begin to delve into your personal behaviour. I'm no behavioural psychologist, body language expert or any other related 'expert', but I am good at using common sense and being aware of people in my surrounding environment. This is exactly what I want you to realise and apply to your life.

I'm being deadly serious when I say that watching and responding to your surroundings is a Jedi skill crucial to your development as a personal trainer. You see, we often wonder why we're not getting clients and why our business ideas are not developing in the way we hoped and expected them to. To change this, we must look through our client's eyes at what they're seeing; we need to assess ourselves.

From this point forward, let's imagine your perfect client. This is the person that you would thrive to working with and who, if given the chance, would form the avatar of 90% of your clientele. What do they want to see in their coach?

The majority of the personal training industry is obsessed with body composition. In many instances, our clients seek some level of improvement to their physique and this is often why a client initially seeks out the help of a trainer, that we know. But the last thing a client wants is to have your ego shoved down their throat. And yet this is often the case in many a gym environment. Have a think about these facets of well-documented behaviour and be 100% honest if you can relate to any of the following:

- Your social media profile picture shows you looking ripped and buff, kitted out in the tightest t-shirt or crop top you can find with every effort being made to look like a magazine cover model
- You wear the tightest top you can find in the gym to flaunt your gains

- You have your post-workout protein shake out on the gym floor to highlight that you've got this fitness lifestyle nailed

- You hang around the front desk or the gym floor with an elitist, often unapproachable demeanour

- You flex your muscles around others at random points, often during conversation, so people can quietly envy your physique

- You never clean the gym equipment because you're better than that

- You make noises in the gym to let others know you lift heavy

- You do the weirdest exercises possible to justify your level of skill, making sure gym members can instantly separate you from the rest of the personal training crowd

- For your workouts, you position yourself in the gym so that everyone can see you, the gym's best personal trainer, in action

How do I know all the above is true?

Because I was guilty of all of this. My actions alienated 90% of the people I wanted to attract into my business. I was arrogant: it was all about me. I used to squat on a swiss ball, make a point of drinking my protein shake in the view of others, avoid or make no effort to clean the gym equipment when asked, parade my elitist persona around the gym, wear the tightest t-shirt I owned, as well as many other embarrassing behaviours that I look back on now with pain.

Remember, people buy off people.

Think back to the last person you looked at in the gym that made you think, 'What a dick'. What was it you disliked about them? A display of gym ego? Always making a point of hogging the most popular piece of kit? Forever making noises as they train? Perhaps they're indirectly doing many of the things you do as a personal trainer, yet often we don't see our own actions. In our own minds, we are the exception. Or perhaps we're simply not self-aware.

Let's be honest and reflect for a moment: is your behaviour attracting or repelling your perfect client? Are you approachable? Do you always have to have others acknowledge your presence? Do you appear arrogant on the gym floor?

If ANY of the above is true in the slightest, you need to address it. People pick up on the smallest aspects of human behaviour.

Truth be told, we are all pretty good at reading the body language of others; for the most part we just don't act on it or are not confident enough in our assumptions to follow up on it. I can tell if someone dislikes me or is just saying words to be polite. I can tell if someone hasn't listened to what I've said or if my actions have annoyed or offended them. Stand back and put yourself in your client's shoes. Would you like what you saw?

Now if your aim is to attract the young alpha fitness buff who wants to weight train, get chicks and become the centre of attention when out at the weekend then by all means display many of the characteristics I mention above. Make yourself known, appear alpha, display your strength and wear that tight t-shirt with pride. But if you're trying to attract everyday people that just want to be healthy, happy, fit, strong and regain their confidence, then reflect on the way you're presenting yourself both physically and in terms of your body language and personal behaviours. Otherwise you're potentially losing out on your ideal client.

Think about the 40 year-old female that wants to get into the gym, gain confidence, lose a few stone and find a manageable way to work out that is enjoyable and not overly time consuming. She doesn't want to eat chicken and broccoli every day to lose weight like the fitness people on Instagram are doing. Are your actions and behaviours going to appeal to her or turn her away?

First impressions count, big time. If I walk into a meeting and if I get a bad vibe about an individual's behaviour, it's likely that I won't work with them or align with them unless all of the following interaction we have during the meeting wins me over and it was just a case of a bad first impression. If you make a bad first impression there is so much work to unwind it that it will likely be a waste of your time. Repeat this behaviour over and over and you will struggle to get clients, grow your gym, or become the success you know you can be.

In my experience how we look and behave is everything. People buy off people.

Think about why you might have chosen to follow my work: what resonated with you? I'm not so smart and professional that I appear boring or overly science-focused. Instead I present myself as approachable, my social media content is unisex, my work is both engaging and inviting and my profile picture depicts a fitness professional without being overly intimidating.

I am me and I make no apologies for that. I try to show the best version of myself every day, treating everyone I meet with respect and never looking to intentionally offend or alienate anyone with what I do or how I act.

I am aware of my audience and act in an appropriate way; you must do the same to be successful at what you do with the people you want to coach. Let's have a think about this stuff now...

Think about your physical appearance...

Are you well presented?

Do you look scruffy or inappropriate?

Do you smell?

Is your hair presentable?

If you have facial hair, is it presentable?

Do your trainers look clean and appropriate for what you do?

X Do you look tired and unhealthy?

Is your t-shirt tucked in?

Are your shorts too short?

Are you appropriately dressed for the situation and environment you're in?

I'm not saying anything above is right or wrong, but you must consider how you want to be viewed by others and be reflective enough to say, "No, Ben's right. I need to change X, Y and Z; it's affecting how people see me and I want to be seen in X way".

This is practicing self-awareness.

I want you to be the best version of yourself in all areas of your life. I want you to have a thriving personal training business or gym and I want you to absolutely love your job with all the satisfaction you have ever dreamed of. And it all starts with you. You are the sales tool; you are the product of your work; you are the 'thing' people are buying from so be sure that your intention matches what people are seeing.

Close this book for a second, we'll come back to these pages. Close your eyes and pick apart all your behaviours and actions that could be improved in order to sky rocket your success as a trainer and reflect on the way in which you can attract your perfect client.

Be honest, be reflective, and identify what needs to change. Not in a week, not next month, now.

Take just 5 minutes to be self-aware, honest, and critical of yourself and let's improve.

Please don't skip this task. I liken this exercise to meditation: people know it's important and despite the big outcome often never do it as the action is so small and seems too 'fluffy' and uncool. It's not what most people do to improve, so why do it?

I hope you are not most people? I want you to be different.

These are some of the actions the world's most successful people do. Reflect, are honest with themselves, learn, and implement change to be better. If not, things never change, and you'll remain a mediocre coach with a mediocre business with mediocre results.

Please ensure that when I ask you to do a task in this book you do it, ideally in a quiet place so you can be calm, think and be in a positon to be truly honest with yourself. Once you have had a think about this, open your eyes and using the next page, write down what you are going to change.

Checklist to change in my behaviour, actions and appearance:

_____

_____

_____

_____

_____

_____

_____

_____

_____

_____

_____

This is also a great task to do as part of your overall personal development. It might make you realise that the character tweaks you're going to make in your professional environment will also become part of your personal environment. Some of those changes come naturally with maturity: I know I improved many of these aspects as I grew older and learned to better understand others. But I know I would have improved so much faster if someone would have pointed them out to me in my earlier years; whether I was in a place to listen at that point in time is another thing. I'd like to think I would have been to the right person, someone I respected and trusted and had seen success in, but who knows. Hindsight is a wonderful thing.

The number of trainers and coaches I talk to who are just not ready to improve and listen is astounding; I'm genuinely gob smacked by this. If a coach approaches me and asks me a question, I will start to respond and explain things to them. Within a matter of seconds, I can see ZERO of what I am saying is going in. Perhaps this is the result of a belief block; they might think they already know what I'm going to say; perhaps they are not ready to change. Perhaps they're just not in a place to absorb information and comprehend it; they might be too tired or too stressed to fully engage in what I'm saying to them. Either way my breath is wasted.

If you are genuinely in a place where you are receptive to advice, are ready for change and want to be the best version of yourself, then this book can teach you profound things.

None of this is rocket science. I am by no means the most knowledgeable man in fitness and nutrition, nor am I the most enlightened. I am, however, in touch with my environment and the people in it. I know what the world is doing; I know how people behave; why people do things and when the words don't match the emotional reality and all I am going to be doing in this book is teaching you a mixture of hard skills to implement, soft skills to try, and realisations or 'ah-ha' moments.

So, if you are with me on this and you're still prepared to be self-aware and improve, I can help you become an AWESOME personal trainer.

Now before you skip to the next chapter, make sure you've completed the above task: it's important.

CHAPTER 2
WALKING THE TALK

As we continue with your personal journey, I want to introduce the idea of walking the talk. Too many coaches are not walking the talk. This doesn't mean looking like a magazine cover model 24/7 and proclaiming that you have the ability to give a client whatever physique they desire.

Put simply, walking the talk is representing yourself as being truly healthy, fit, happy, well-presented and an inspiration to others. Remember this: you should be the inspiration for your clients. So again, let's raise some questions about where you are at:

Do you sleep poorly and does it show in your appearance and work ethic?

Are you practicing a lifestyle and eating in a manner that you promote to your clients?

Are you the under-recovered personal trainer always carrying a coffee cup and relying on caffeine in order to function?

Are you full of energy? Would your clients consider you fun to be around? Or are you a bit of a bore because you're always tired with no real interest in your clients' needs?

Does your teaching inspire and show clients you truly care for their needs?

Does your appearance fit the context of your sport or gym practices?

Do you have an attainable, maintainable appearance that others might consider healthy?

Are you strong and able to practice the skills you teach your clients?

Chapter 1 focused on the behaviour side of what we do as coaches; now I want to focus on the way we look and perform as people. If we're constantly tired, run down, yawning and not walking the talk of our trade, then how do we hope to inspire our clients?

Remember, people are very receptive to body language. If your body language, movement capabilities, performance and overall appearance don't match what you are teaching, then not only are you are a hypocrite, you will not have the success you desire. Clients will feed off your energy, your abilities and the way you present yourself; they're likely to progress to a standard that's ultimately the result of your actions. If the client sees you as the epitome and the professional, are you providing them with the potential to challenge their own abilities and be the best version of themselves?

If you are drinking coffee to always stay alert and awake and feel normal, your clients will view this as a standard practice.

If you don't take care of your own health and fitness, the chances are your clients won't push themselves to their true potential. You set their standard of what is considered healthy and achievable; if you don't then why should they do otherwise.

If you skip the movement and flexibility portion of your training to focus solely on the heavier strength work then your clients will also apply this mindset to their training. Remember, you set the standards, starting with yourself: your walk and your actions, not your talk.

Let's imagine you're teaching your client a hip flexor stretch. You drop down into a demonstration of the stretch and complain that your hip flexor feels tight. You then tell your client, "Actually, that feels pretty tight on me, I should stretch more". What does that tell the client in this instance?

Yes you've demonstrated the stretch, but whether you realise it or not you've highlighted that stretching's not that important. Through your actions, your client will subconsciously be thinking, "Well you evidently don't stretch enough, but you can still walk, squat and do your workouts without any trouble. I'm pretty sure I can get away without stretching. I'd rather just get to the real work. If that's what you do, then I can do that too".

It's not in your clients' interests to know whether your hip flexors are tight or not. Ideally, you should move well and be a product of your training services. Your body should reflect the vision of health and fitness you teach, but if not, don't parade it to your client. Yes that might seem a little dishonest, but you have to consider the message you're sending out to them. In the above situation, you're not highlighting the importance of stretching for your workouts; if it's not that important to you, it's not going to be a priority for them.

People want to do the bare minimum to succeed in anything; it's just human nature.

Your clients may have been doing the bare minimum their whole life to lose weight. Whether that be as a result of crappy diets, minimal workouts at home or taking the newest weight-loss pills. They want short cuts. By failing to walk your talk you've just highlighted another issue to them without even knowing it.

Like I've said, people pick up on a surprising amount of information and if they can do the bare minimum needed to achieve some form of result, they will. Your clients may not yet fully understand or appreciate why mobility is an important pre-requisite to the squat, but you've just given them another reason to question improving their movement. You've shown it's not that important to you. Your client senses that too.

The way we present ourselves and how that reflects on the advice we give our clients is everything. Every detail counts.

Let's start with you: what do you need to improve on?

Your sleep?

Your movement?

Your diet and what you are eating?

Your energy and love for your job around your clients?

Your body composition? *(over time) learning process*

✱ Your ability to demonstrate an exercise confidently? ✱

Whatever it is, it's time to make another list. I want you to make a list of 3-5 key things you're going to personally work on to be an inspiration to others and walk the talk. Turn over the page and make your list and next to each item, explain how you are going to do it and what you need to change to get there.

First thing to change:

_____

Habits or actions to implement and achieve your first change:

_____

_____

_____

_____

Second thing to change:

_____

Habits or actions to implement and achieve your second change:

_____

_____

_____

_____

Third thing to change:

_____

Habits or actions to implement and achieve your third change:

_____

_____

_____

_____

Fourth thing to change:

_____

Habits or actions to implement and achieve your fourth change:

_____

_____

_____

_____

Fifth thing to change:

_____

Habits or actions to implement and achieve your fifth change:

_____

_____

_____

_____

Struggling for ideas?

Here's an example:

First thing to change:

Get more sleep so I am more alert and present with my clients

Habits or actions to implement and achieve your first change:

1. Get to sleep by 10.00pm so I am fresh when I wake up at 6.00am
2. Turn my phone off at 9.30pm so I have no sleep distractions
3. Finish with clients at 9pm so I can keep on top of my sleep
4. Don't drink coffee past 4pm so it doesn't interfere with my sleep

At this point if you think you need help with your diet, lifestyle and changing your body composition, visit the shop at www.bodytypenutrition.co.uk or at my website www.bencoomber.com and grab a copy of 'The Nutrition Blueprint', my book about optimising your diet and lifestyle. After all, it starts with you. If you don't feel you have the knowledge to make these changes, acquire it then apply it.

I need you to walk the talk.

We need to optimise you first before we can truly optimise your clients.

Be the inspiration you hoped you always would be to your clients.

P.S. No turning the page until you've done the exercise.

CHAPTER 3
TALKING TO CLIENTS

The next stage in client communication is the art of talking to your clients, both in person and online. Having discussed the role of body language in communication, let's now focus on the more direct approaches we can take to ensure your client feels valued, cared for and understands the reasoning behind your chosen coaching processes that will lead them towards their goals.

In-person communication

There's a trend amongst trainers in the fitness industry to always be right. I see it online all the time and I've been guilty of it in the past with my clients. I'd try and prove how clever I was to my clients and to other trainers by using big words and being scientifically correct about everything.

In reality, 95% of your clients won't understand or care about the minor details that form a large part of many an online feud. The key message here is to talk your client's language: convey your message to them in the most simple and meaningful way possible. Confuse them with scientific jargon and the chances are, whatever you wanted to achieve will never be accomplished.

Here is a classic example:

The word 'tone' is widely understood by a large section of the population. It's been used by the media, personal trainers and throughout fitness marketing for decades. If I speak about 'toning up', the majority of people would understand what I mean. It's an effective term that roughly translates in people's minds to losing some fat, creating some shape and revealing some muscle to improve overall improved body composition.

However, delve into the depths of the internet and it won't take long before you find a group of people furiously shaking their science wands, arguing that the term 'tone' has no real meaning. Regardless of what the official concept should say or imply, for the most part, it doesn't matter. There is zero point in me explaining to my client that the term 'tone' doesn't mean what we think it does. Your client doesn't care. They just want to sculpt their glutes and find the most effective way to achieve this.

Talk your client's language.

Yes we might have a lot of scientific know-how and be aware of the correct terminology for things that are important within our industry, but how much does it really matter. We're not achieving anything by having internet debates about the correct way to explain a process. We're ultimately aiming to get our client to perform an action that helps them reach a specific goal.

Simply put, our clients just want results.

There are instances when this concept changes: if you work with a client over time, you might choose to layer more information on them as they become more experienced and hungry for knowledge. But in the early stages, especially in the first 3-6 months of their journey, keep your message simple and don't overcomplicate things. Over time if your client becomes curious and wants to be educated, and then by all means teach them the finer details. But be sure to pick this time wisely.

The subject of pain is a common area in which explanations are often complicated and lost on the client. Let's say a client feels pain in their scapular region and you know it's a referred pain from their rhomboids or supraspinatus; don't bombard them with the anatomy. Instead, let your client know your thoughts by using visual cues and touch to explain your reasoning. Your client will understand what you're telling them and having made sense of the information, will be more likely to follow any advice you then give them.

Speak their language; keep it simple and understandable where possible, using terms your clients know ('tone', 'shoulder' etc).

Reading body language and adjusting your speech

Remember, every client is different. If I was a coaching a 40-year-old female who has been feeling overworked, stressed and dedicates a large portion of her life to her children, then be receptive to her needs. Be aware of her character traits, listen to her frustrations and note changes in her body language and adjust the way you behave and speak accordingly. In this instance, you might speak quieter, have less dominance in your posture, use your hands when talking (it's easier to trust someone if you can see their hands) and try to mirror her actions as much as possible.

This doesn't mean you are not firm as a coach when you need to be, sometimes this is highly warranted and needed, especially with this character type that might make a lot of excuses about their lack of progression, but you adapt how you speak and hold yourself in the early contact stages with your client to make her more receptive to the time you are going to spend with one another.

On the other hand, if my client was a young rugby player with a laddish character who doesn't take himself too seriously, again I would adjust yourself accordingly. Crack a joke here and there, stand with a bit more dominance in your posture, speak with a little more slang.

Always adjust your behaviour to suit your client.

This isn't throwing Chapter 1 out of the window. You're still being professional and presenting yourself well, but by adapting your language to that of the client (or prospective client) you will build rapport quicker and your client will be more responsive to your ideas. This also doesn't mean pretending to be someone different or acting out of character. Rather, you're making a few small tweaks to put yourself on the same level as your client.

There will always be people that you won't connect with, and that's ok. If you find yourself in this situation, don't stress. You're not going to be a perfect fit for everyone. And if you do push ahead and take on a client regardless of your concerns, then it's possible that you'll struggle to get results. Building rapport will be difficult and neither you or your client will enjoy the coaching/client relationship.

We've all experienced THAT client: you don't have a lot to talk about, conversation is a struggle and everything feels a little awkward. In this instance, be honest and remove yourself from the situation. You need to enjoy coaching all your clients and if you know this relationship is going to be a struggle, I'd recommend you focus on the people that you can connect with and who will truly benefit from your training.

That being said, while this person in question may not be appropriate for 1-2-1 sessions, semi-private or group training may be a better fit for them. There are always options to best suit the client's needs, always be mindful of this. We'll discuss this in more detail later on.

Online communication

Face-to-face won't be your only dealings with clients; there will be emails, texts, Whatsapp messages, Facebook messages and more. How you talk through online communication is just as important as speaking in-person.

Going back to my two previous examples (the 40-year-old female and the young rugby player), your approach to both will, and should, be different. If your usual texting style is full of emojis and kisses and the relationship with your client is appropriate to use that, then by all means be you and use that approach. But be mindful that this style of communication won't fit with everyone and in some cases, you may have to be more professional and use different language.

With that being said, don't act one way in person and another way on-line. Your style of language and the way you communicate needs to be the same wherever possible. Consistency is key; a lack of consistency will breed a lack of trust and may be enough to make a client question their trust in you. Always be consistent.

Setting your boundaries

When working with clients, it's important to set boundaries. Too many coaches have an open-door policy of 'text me anytime' and 'If you need me, just contact me'. This is the catalyst for a poor work-life balance and feeling tied to your needier clients. Remember that you oversee the relationship with your clients, so set the lines of communication from day 1.

When I coach someone online I am very clear with my processes. With every client I have a set procedure in place as follows:

1. Monday is the day I check in on your client folder. Thus please update your Dropbox folder over the weekend and ensure I have everything I'll need in there as requested

2. Email me with your questions and I will reply with all the needed information and adjustments based on your uploaded files

3. I am here for small things on Whatsapp and will reply during my normal working hours of 7am-4pm via Whatsapp, text or voice message

4. If we have a Skype chat as part of your package, your feedback and questions will be carried out on a Monday night or at the time we set for your Skype coaching call

5. Results and major adjustments should be made weekly. Small changes made over Whatsapp are fine, but only expect replies during working hours

And that's my coaching set up: plain and simple with clear boundaries. Then all I do is schedule in ½ a day or a full day depending on client demands and volume and on Monday I sit down and do all my primary coaching on that day.

Clear process, and allocate time in my diary to get it done.

In my above example I've been firm but fair to my clients. I've set them clear working times and they know when they have access to my coaching time. I've also outlined the most effective ways for them to communicate with me. My clients are still being provided for: they're still being kept accountable and they know what data I need from them to do my job effectively. Furthermore, it allows me the time I need to maintain a good work-life balance. I don't want to be answering client calls at 9pm when they're looking for advice on food to buy for dinner.

We all need space and it's important to set up boundaries for your business. If there's a lack of contact from you for the service they're paying you for, then that's completely unacceptable. However, if you have been clear on outlining your availability and the service they're paying for, your requests are completely justified.

Remember that it's up to you to decide on your working relationship, not the client.

If this is the first time you've set clear boundaries with a client then it can be difficult for some to adjust to your new schedule. As long as you inform them of the changes through a well-mannered email or a friendly chat in person, there should be no issues.

For example, if you are sending out an email or group Whatsapp, you might write something like this:

Dear Jane,

I just wanted to reach out to you and explain a few changes I'm making to my schedule in order to provide you with a better personal training service.

I've been too available to my clients and need to manage my working hours a little more effectively from here on in. This will give me the time I need to focus on delivering you the best possible personal training service as we work on reaching your goals.

I feel that the following guidelines will allow us to continue working together as smoothly as possible:

Training sessions and appointments will be organised in person at a time when we both have our diaries at hand. If this is not possible, arrangements can then be made by text and I will reply during my normal working hours of 7-5pm to schedule your session

Please text me if have any queries but don't expect a reply between the hours of 8pm and 9am

Please bring your food diary to your Monday session and we will discuss it during the last 10 minutes of the session as we cool down rather than picking this up in parts throughout the week via text

Please keep your weekly progress tracker up-to-date in your Dropbox folder and continue to upload your progress photos every 4 weeks

I really appreciate your help on this as it would mean so much to me to get this working and moving forward. Should you have any questions then I'm more than happy to chat about them at our next session.

Regards.

Coach.

When corresponding with your own clients, the points mentioned above may not fit with your business model or the way in which you operate. The example above is there to be used as a guide: adapt it as required for your needs.

When making changes to your schedule, don't feel that you need to justify your reasons or explain that you need to gain more control of your free time. Be firm and set boundaries, make the request and inform your clients of the changes. There's no reason to make apologies for your business decisions.

Own your decisions and be the person in control; don't be afraid of outlining your chosen rules. Your work life balance is crucial as you become a more effective trainer, and setting boundaries in a manner that your clients understand and resonate with will facilitate your success.

Ongoing communication

Talking to your client in a session may seem like an obvious form of communication, but I want to focus in on the initial requirements you set them at the beginning of their fitness journey.

It's often tempting to brush over the basics of health and get to the advanced discussions on carb cycling and ergogenic aids. Regardless of your expertise or the demands from your client to rush through the fitness basics, it's your professional duty as a trainer to regularly question their sleep cycles, daily hydration and dietary patterns. Over time those basic daily practices will become habitual. After all, it's the basics that form the foundational steps on the path to success.

Diligently addressing keys concepts such as sleep, hydration and protein intake will also allow you to spot potential lifestyle issues that consistently cause problems for your client. You can tell a client to sleep more and improve their quality of sleep, but how do they put that into practice? You might have explained a few techniques that could be beneficial, but your client may need further help in implementing your ideas into their life and pre-existing commitments. Change is never easy and every client is going to have his or her reasons for struggling to change: a problematic partner, health concerns, children, an addiction to Netflix, work commitments, social occasions...I could go on.

Life is full of obstacles that result in excuses to avoid change. It's ESSENTIAL that you keep revisiting this information and working out alternative strategies to challenge and hopefully overcome the hindrances. Don't feel bad for nagging your clients if they don't follow up on advice. Remember it's your job to help them change their lifestyle. That's what they're paying you for!

With that in mind, be curious and enquire often about their lifestyle habits:

How did you sleep last night?

What did you eat for breakfast this morning?

Did you drink enough water yesterday?

Each time a client responds with a 'no', there's a reason they couldn't do what was asked of them. Here is your opportunity to delve deeper and find a solution to work around the problem. The more you talk and discuss the roadblocks, the greater the relationship you build with your client and the more likely you are to create long-lasting change.

And remember what we discussed in Chapter 2: scrutinise and assess your own habits. If you're not getting those basics right yourself, you'll be unable to communicate your ideas successfully to your clients.

Be the example. Be the leader and walk the talk.

Then when you do talk, set the boundaries, be clear in the expectations from your relationship, and always get on their level where possible.

CHAPTER 4
ASKING WHY

We're taking our communication skills from Chapter 3 and implementing them in our next step to becoming the AWESOME personal trainers we all have the potential to be. It's time to talk about goal setting.

It's a scene I'm sure you're all familiar with:

"Sarah, I want you to tell me your goals. What do you want to achieve from your sessions with me?"

"Well Ben, I'd like to lose weight and feel better. I guess I'd like to have some more energy"

We've assessed Sarah's goals and they seem to be both legitimate and realistic. Done. She's looking for weight loss so let's get to it.

Or should we probe further?

The goals that Sarah has described will have formed the backdrop of her goals for years. Except she's never achieved them. Sarah is always aiming to 'lose weight' but she never seems to complete the task.

Maybe she doesn't try hard enough?

Putting our judgements aside and asking her to elaborate, Sarah then starts to talk about her life. She's been on a diet for years, in fact, she's never off dieting. And diets are just the beginning: she's bought an endless number of home workouts, she's tried the 'health' foods, the skinny teas and the weight loss shakes. If there's the potential to lose weight by doing a workout or eating a certain food, Sarah has trialled them all.

What were her previous goals in each of the above situations:

"Oh I still had the same goals. I wanted to lose weight and feel better. And I wanted to have more energy"

So, what's going to change this time around? What's going to motivate your client to modify their lifestyle with your guidance? If Sarah was your client and you set her a plan based on the vague hope of 'losing weight' with no real context, are you confident of her success? Chances are she's likely to fail and add personal training to the list of weight loss failures that cost her money and didn't work.

Why is Sarah not achieving her goals?

You'll find the answer and the key to her success within that sentence: WHY.

It's not uncommon to train clients who don't have a powerful reason for change. They know they should have a goal in mind, but the goal they tell the trainer doesn't truly resonate with their innermost desires or needs. Most of the time clients don't know why they want to change; perhaps part of that reason boils down to the client not truly understanding their own whys, or perhaps they haven't yet realised their why. And it's up to you to find out.

How many people do you know who want to lose weight? I reckon if I asked 100 people off the street, 80-90 of those people would say they wanted to achieve some form of weight loss. On face value people want to change, but that change isn't happening. Why?

Because the why doesn't ignite a fire within them to spark change.

I could be jumping the gun here, but if your client tells you they'd like to lose weight, feel better and have some more energy, they'll have a why in some form or other. Everyone will have their own individual reasons for change and for losing weight but sometimes it's hard.

Discussing reasons can be challenging in itself and oftentimes scary; we don't talk about our feelings and modern society doesn't allow us to be open with how we feel. It's often seen as being selfish or weak; who are we to burden others with our problems? Clients may not have developed enough trust to open up to us and discuss their personal life. Especially not in front of a young, sprightly personal trainer who's the epitome of physical perfection.

Before you sit down with a new client and discuss their diet, training plan, lifestyle habits and supplements, it's important to address some form of goal setting process based on their whys.

And if you want profound change in your client, you have to dig to a deeper emotional level. The answers you find will form the foundations that will shape your client's journey. The why is the ignition to power them into making the right choices when the rest of the world is telling them to order a burger and eat cake. We need the whys to create more powerful pushes for our clients when the world is pulling them in.

Push vs pull

Every day your client is faced with decisions: environmental decisions and social pressures from those around them to be the norm. To do as they've always done, regardless of the consequences.

Sarah is at work. It's Friday and Friday is cake day in the office. Sarah has a decision to make: are her reasons to avoid eating the cake more powerful than her reasons to tuck in like everyone else?

If she was following her original goal:

"I'd like to lose weight and feel better. I guess I'd like to have some more energy"

Could cake make her feel better? Everyone likes cake.

"Ah forget the plan, it's only one slice of cake. It will be ok, I'll try have a light dinner. If not I'll get back on it tomorrow"

Yet tomorrow never comes in reality, every day a client will be presented with these decisions, to eat the cake or not, to drink or not, to have the burger or not, to do the right thing or not.

It's our aim as personal trainers to empower Sarah into reaching her goals from the power of her personal why. If we can do that, then the push is stronger than the pull. There is real emotion and a genuine reason for her to confidently say 'NO' in her choices.

If you find yourself in a similar situation with a client like Sarah who has come to you with vague weight loss aims, ask why, then why again. Gather a list of reasons that your client feels emotionally attached to and charged up about. You'll have provided them with a newly focused vision and an appreciation for why they're doing what you've asked of them.

How you approach the why will vary amongst different clients. You may choose to enquire through silence and patience, giving your client the time to talk and let them explain why they really want to achieve what they do. Now I say silence for a reason. Too many personal trainers feel awkward in silence. They ask a question, there's an awkward silence for a second or two and your client feels uncomfortable. We start talking to fill the awkward silence and help them out and ultimately put words in their mouth. If you want to get to the bottom of your client's personal motivators, then you must stop doing this. Learn to be comfortable with silence.

Your client should and needs to feel uncomfortable. They haven't been forced to go to a place like this before, and that should instantly show you that this exercise is key to behavioural change.

Learn to be comfortable with awkward silences between you and your clients. This is where the magic comes from; when we build on our relationships, we get a truly honest why. Be patient and wait as long as possible for your client to come up with their reasons. This process might take time and you might have to probe into some dark places, but its vitally important to get there in the end.

Reasons for change will be varied and everyone is unique. Don't be surprised or shocked by a client's why. Here are some examples of drivers for change that are genuine to many of the clients you will have. Yes some of these might shock you, but this is real life, a real insight into your clients mind and how most of us actually think:

"When I take my clothes off I want my partner to be sexually attracted to me again. I know he isn't. I've put on 5 stone and really let myself go"

"I want to be able to take off my clothes and not be disgusted with myself. I've had enough, this has to change"

"I wear baggy clothes and always wear black just to try and look slimmer than I am. I want to be happy with my body and stop hiding it away"

"I want to be able to run around the park with my kids and not get out of breath after 2 minutes. I used to be so fit, my level of fitness is an embarrassment"

"I want to be a healthy example to my kids. I'm sick of being the fat dad, I want my kids to feel proud of me"

"I'm fed up of my fat jiggling when I walk up the stairs. And let's not get started on how it feels when I try run up the stairs, that's if my knees don't hurt!"

"I want to be able to fit into all my nice clothes again. I've got half a wardrobe of size 12 clothing going to waste"

"I want to feel alive every day and be happy, healthy and energised. I've not felt like that for 10 years. I'm always tired, lethargic and fed up of life"

"I want my libido back. I've not had a decent sex life with my partner for years and we've drifted apart because of it. We're just companions and I don't want that. I want us to lust after one another like we did when we were younger"

Many of those reasons will sound extremely personal but this is the reality of why people want to change. At 18 when I was on my own weight loss journey I had my own whys:

"If I don't lose weight I will be unsuccessful in my career. I want success. I don't want to be that fat jolly actor that everyone laughs at who always ends up playing the funny role"

"I want to be sexually attractive to women so I can someday get a girlfriend"

"I want to have real confidence, not the fake confidence I get from acting. Everyone thinks I'm confident but deep down I'm not"

"I don't want to be ill and struggle with my IBS and eczema any longer; I want to feel energised and healthy"

I was seriously attached to my whys. Notice the difference between the examples and our 'lose weight and feel better' goal at the beginning of this chapter.

For me my whys were so much more than that. Yes I wanted to lose weight and get healthy, but why. I had powerful and genuine reasons behind what I was doing that drove me every day to make the right choices: to hit the gym when I was meant to, to eat the right foods, say no to the cake and some meals out, get to bed on time, ensure I drank enough water and have stronger reasons to push away the negative parts of my environment that was continually trying to pull me in.

Question your clients and ask them 'Why?' Be patient and wait out the awkward silence; probe and get to the bottom of things and explain to them that this process is paramount to creating powerful enough reasons to change, despite how uncomfortable and vulnerable they feel doing this. Failure to do this will get your clients the same old lacklustre results they always do. Get better results, get deeper and closer to your whys.

Blocking factors to change

When a person is seeking change there will be legitimate environmental blocking factors pulling them hard in the opposite direction. There will be times when it's really difficult to say no, especially when that blocking factor is a loved one or a habitual action they've been doing for years and half the time don't even know they are doing it.

A problematic partner is a classic example. A partner might encourage nights out for dinner, social drinks and a variety of self-indulgent habits that, as a couple, have been the norm for years. Take the time and talk through these problems with your clients. It's important to chat through strategies and different techniques for them to try in order to build the confidence to approach these difficult conversations with the people they love. Your client may then choose to sit their partner down and work out the issues in an amicable and supportive fashion:

"Clive, I want to change, and I need your support. I'm really trying to lose weight and I'm finding it hard when we keep drinking during the week and going out at weekends for indulgent meals. It's not helping me to lose the weight.

I get that you enjoy the meals and the drinks, so do I, but I'd really like more support from you. I don't want you to make me feel guilty for saying no to going out for dinner, or choosing a healthier place to eat, or making me feel bad for not drinking.

It would be amazing if you came on this journey with me to lose some weight and get healthier too. We can still do things together but I understand if you don't feel like being a part of it. All I ask is that you support me as I try to achieve this for myself and I need to change some habits in our lifestyle to achieve this".

It's not an easy conversation to have. Clients might feel as though they're pushing their partner away or looking to place blame for the way they feel. Or perhaps they're not used to being this honest with their partner.

But as their personal trainer, you must address these issues with your client and put them in a place where they feel confident to have these conversations. Support your client, get to the root cause of the issues and empower them with strategies to overcome the difficult stages. That's when the true magic happens.

The coaching process and standing your ground

Throughout the coaching process you have to stand your ground and continue to highlight key reasons why your clients aren't getting the results they want if they're not doing what's required of them. Be firm.

If your client comes in every week and complains about a lack of results and you know it's because their old habits are creeping in, be firm and don't be too quick to offer other solutions. Whether it's going out at the weekends, being too indulgent or eating too many calories, address the lack of accountability on the client's part. They need to accept they're at fault here.

If we use the example of a client eating too much, keep highlighting that issue as you review their plan and find ways for them to address the glaring problem that's needing to be resolved. The client has to know where you stand with your advice and what they need to change to get the results they're looking for. Only when they're ready to accept this and if it's necessary, can you then offer alternative interventions.

Remember, there are no short cuts; stand your ground and address the problems.

Throughout your coaching process ensure you are probing, talking and helping a client with their problems and blocking factors. They will know why they need more sleep or what they need to eat less of. Be real and don't be afraid to get personal.

Probe, be honest and find out why. Find direct solutions to their problems, and client success will be yours.

CHAPTER 5
ASSESSING YOUR CLIENT

Assessing your client is an important process. But do you have to sit them down right at the beginning and talk through everything? Is there a step by step process we have to deliver every time?

Time and time again in the world of health and fitness, there is a frustrating concept that we use to answer questions most of the time...

...context.

Never underestimate the importance of context. There are times where we crave an answer to a problematic or difficult scenario and throughout your career you'll be asked many different questions and be expected to come up with a generalised, easy to implement, answer. But expect many answers to begin with something along the lines of, "Well, it all depends on the context".

Annoying. But it's the truth.

Sometimes an answer requires many a pre-requisite. Often we have to take the client's age, height, weight, environment, beliefs, support structure, movement ability, knowledge of nutrition and family history into consideration. And depending on what your question is will determine what factors back up your answer.

It's not uncommon to hear a personal trainer wanting answers for a client that begins along the lines of: "My client is not losing weight. She's eating well, moving well, sleep pretty decent but what's going wrong?"

To provide guidance, we could hypothesise lots of different answers or reasons; but to get close to the best answer first time, we would want to explore the context. In doing so, we can take into account other factors that might be affecting the client's lack of results.

As a personal trainer, there are many processes we go through when dealing with a client. People are complicated. Their problems are multi-faceted and it's our job to sit down and make it as simple as humanly possible for them, which is why the answer to a problem is rarely black and white.

What should you ask?

As I've previously discussed, one of the key reasons why people don't change is because they're overwhelmed at the prospect of overhauling every aspect of their lives. It's a lot of work. Only when you understand the thought processes going on in your client's head can you then start to truly help them. Many of your clients won't think like a fitness professional, so how do we circumnavigate this in the assessment process?

What you assess and what you're looking to change will depend entirely on your client's readiness to change and their goals.

Let's come back to Tom Cowan whom I spoke of in the introduction. He was one of the people on my journey who made me realise I had to work on my people skills as a personal trainer. Tom's initial client assessment was pretty basic, never more than 10-15 minutes of a sit down with the client. I, on the other hand, would talk to my clients for 60-90 minutes on that initial assessment prior to any training. Tom would do a Par-Q, run through some basic measurements and set some basic goals and targets for his clients. Within the first session they would be out on the gym floor on the treadmill, just chatting before going on to do some form of training. Our assessments both covered the essentials (in the clients mind), but I liked to carry out a nutritional assessment, a full movement screen and discuss multiple goals and primary drivers of change. I liked to cover all sorts and I was thorough in my assessment process.

Which assessment process is correct?

Both.

It's all about the context.

Being in the commercial gym environment, I think Tom's process was far more suitable for the clients of that particular gym at first contact, or especially in the early phases of the coach / client relationship. They weren't overwhelmed with information and homework that made them feel like being back at school.

He did some basic testing, outlined some goals, then started immediately with their training. He was doing what he was paid to do: get clients fit and losing weight. My approach focused on a lifestyle overhaul. For many it was complex and rather tedious. This was at a time when my methods were producing 20-30% success, 40% at a push on a good month. Tom was killing it and his approach was about as simple as it could get.

So, how simple should our assessment process be? And how much information do we give out at the beginning?

Here it comes again... it's all about the context!

We need to decide what stage the client is at on their journey before we take any further action. Tom worked that information out over a couple of sessions just by getting to know the client. Tom would have the client on the treadmill for 10-15 minutes chatting, warming up and getting the blood flowing. He'd then move them through squatting, throwing and moving; nothing technical, but introducing them to the format of a workout. Throughout the session and over weeks that followed, he'd be chatting, exploring, watching their movement and assessing the behaviours of his clients. During that time Tom was building rapport, developing trust and learning about the client's character and mindset while helping them to move better and become fitter.

Is this the right approach for your clients?

Only you can decide that. Personally, I think that Tom's technique works well in a commercial gym environment as a starting point for the coach / client relationship and their expectations of working with a PT early doors.

But regardless of my opinions at this point, you must treat every client like a unique snowflake and try gauge how 'hard-core' to start them off. What are they ready for? Where is their head at? What do they expect from you as a coach?

Let's use a different scenario to add more context to this situation. Let's say I own a gym, or I'm a trainer in a small studio. The reasons for a client choosing my smaller facility over a commercial gym will be different. In this situation, the client may already be in a higher state of change and has chosen to seek training in a private facility for more focused training time. As it's a more personal environment, a client is likely to expect a more thorough training and nutrition assessment. There's an expectation of an attentive service here and we should change our approach to match that expectation.

It's important to recognise that expectation can be a dangerous thing and can negatively affect your business relations. One person expects one outcome, you give them another and they become frustrated when the money they've spent hasn't delivered the outcome they had hoped for. Instances like this highlight the importance of knowing your client and having the skill to address any issues when they arise. It can be useful to ask about expectations in your pre-qualification process. You can then use this information to guide your client's sessions.

If at any point you need to change your approach, knowing that any alterations may not align with the client's original expectations, talk to your client and be honest with them. Explain the reasons for change and allow the client to appreciate why such changes are necessary. If you go ahead and change things without their knowledge, then it's understandable why the client would feel annoyed.

Everything in life can be solved with greater communication. If we can get off on the right foot with all of our clients, then we stand an infinitely better chance of long term success with them.

So which approach is right for you?

Again, only you can decide that. Think about your gym environment and the people in it: think about their personalities, training habits and their general approaches to life. Think about your price point, your experience, your abilities and the client's expectations from your format of personal training. Having taken all of this into consideration, you will be able to determine the correct assessment process for their wants and needs based on the background information you've acquired.

Both Tom and I had the correct approaches to our assessment. Tom's approach was more appropriate for the environment we were in; mine wasn't. I had come from working in a studio where the expected approach was more detailed and in-depth. Our commercial gym was different: clients wanted to come in and move, they wanted to be trained while feeling healthier and losing weight. They didn't care too much for my deeply analytical assessments, too few were ready for that.

Like I said, it's all about the context.

The importance of communication

As I've mentioned previously, I'm a very reflective person: I always like to reflect on my experiences as an opportunity to better my abilities and the delivery of my skills. There is one particular example that sticks out in my mind as a turning point for change.

I had been flyering in my local area for the studio I was based in at the time. The studio itself was part of a small business park that had approximately 50 other businesses based there. It was the perfect hunting ground for potential clients. I created a flyer detailing my role at the studio with a call to action that would hopefully get people in the door. I dropped a flyer around every business, asking them to put it up in a communal area or share it around the office. Two days later, I went around the offices and asked if the flyer had been passed around and if anyone had any questions.

Within a few days a lady walked in to the studio enquiring about my personal training services for her husband as a birthday present. I talked her through what I had to offer and gave her a price for 10 sessions including a free assessment and massage to kick-start his training. When her husband came in, we carried out his initial assessment and we were ready to start. I had money in the bank for his 10 sessions and had bagged myself a new client. I was ecstatic!

But my approach was catastrophic. From the moment money exchanged hands, the coach/client relationship was doomed to fail.

You see, this particular client wasn't ready for change; it was his wife that had sought out my services. He also had no previous experience of being in a gym environment. His idea of a training session was to arrive, move around, get the job done and leave as quickly as possible. So of course I went against all his pre-conceived ideas and gave him everything, he got the works. I looked at his movement, his nutrition, his lifestyle habits, his readiness for change; we covered it all. And to be fair, he stuck with me for 5 sessions.

One day he approached me to tell me what I didn't want to hear: "Ben, I won't be training with you today. I'd like to cancel the rest of my sessions and get a refund for my remaining sessions with you".

I was devastated. Not least because I'd already spent the money on my rent and I was barely earning a liveable wage as it was. I asked him what made him decide to cancel his sessions and he told me everything I did wrong.

"When I started training with you I just wanted to get fit and I was excited at the time. This would be the starting point for me finally getting fit after letting myself go for so long. But I didn't think it would be so intense with all the assessments, the nutrition, the stuff at home, there's just so much to change.

But my biggest issue is with the sessions. We're just not doing anything. We spend nearly 40 minutes of my session stretching and I came here to get fit, I don't want to stretch. I know I'm tight and I do need to improve my flexibility, but I also want to lose weight and get fit. That hasn't happened at all in the last month. So, I'd like a refund please. I wish you all the best for the future but this isn't for me".

The most heart-breaking thing for me writing this now, and something that has stayed in my mind for years, is that I had the power to change this guy's life. Instead I didn't address his basic needs and may have potentially put him off fitness for life.

We have power in our hands as personal trainers. Great power. We can use that power to inspire people or put them off training for life. I fear that my approach to helping this particular client gave him the impression that fitness is too much of an effort. That it's all hard work. That a session in the gym requires 40 minutes of stretching before you even think about working out; that you can't eat carbs at X times and to feel fitter requires a complete lifestyle overhaul.

I'm here to inspire people, not to scare and alienate them as they work on becoming fit and healthy. And yet as an industry we seem oblivious to the reality in which we alienate everyday people from our world: posting endless selfies of our ripped abs and our weekly food prep, telling clients that they 'don't want it badly enough' and boasting about how much of our time is spent dedicated to our physiques.

You get the idea here. We are part of the problem. The more we promote the unachievable lifestyle, the harder we make it look. It's not inspiring people to change, it's turning them away.

And as an industry we need to come together and stand up for simplicity.

As a side note, if you have no idea what actually goes through the head of your average client, the problems they face, what it takes them to get fit and healthy, and what they think of the industry and of trainers, ask them, I think you'll be shocked.

In my earlier days as a trainer, I didn't want to show simplicity; I used to worry about what other trainers thought of me. I wanted to show that I was the best; I had to be seen as the elite and I had to present my knowledge in a way that demonstrated I could train people far better and with more complexity than anyone else in the gym.

In reality, it doesn't matter what others think. Comparing and trying to prove yourself is stopping you from being a great trainer and helping the people that really matter: your clients. Your clients are the people paying for your services, no one else. The opinions of the female trainer you're trying to impress, other gym members and the management team don't pay your wage. If you focus your energy on being attentive to the needs of your paying clients, it will show. The genuine belief and connection that comes as a result of the sessions you deliver to them are the impressions that matter the most to the outside world.

Coming back to my unhappy client, what should I have done to improve the level of success I had with him?

I should have been more Tom.

I should have kept things simple and carried out a basic assessment and got him moving. I should have guided him through some beginner stretches between rest periods and challenged his cardiovascular endurance which tied in with his aims to improve his general fitness. I shouldn't have bombarded him with knowledge, instead discussing food tips or lifestyle improvements in the last 5-10 minutes of each session. All those improvements would have him moving towards his goal while I layered snippets of valuable information to him in smaller chunks, chunks he could handle. Had this been my initial plan then perhaps he'd have completed his 10 training sessions and felt proud of his achievements. If I matched my client's expectations, then I could have helped him achieve his goals and potentially continued training with him beyond his initial 10 sessions.

Instead I scared him off. He cancelled his remaining sessions and I had to give a refund. I have to live with the fact I might have put someone off of their quest to better their health. Personally, that's a hard thing for me. But on reflection it's taught me a valuable lesson: care for the needs of your clients. Always.

Back to assessing your client

I hope that my experiences have given you an idea of the processes we have to consider for that all-important client assessment process.

1. Listen to your client. Get chatting. Find out what they want to achieve and deliver it to them in the simplest way possible. Be present, listen and don't allow your assumptions to alter your perception of their needs. Refuse to acknowledge the needs of your client and you risk damaging your training relationship for good

2. Understand their expectations from you and don't be afraid to ask them what they want from you and from their training sessions. Aligning their expectations with yours from day 1 allows you to develop a positive training relationship

3. Avoid information overload. While this isn't always an easy task to get right, aim for a middle ground between educating your client and overkill. Be aware that experience plays a role in getting the balance right; nurturing a relationship is a skill that takes time to master

4. Build rapport and layer complex information to your client over time as their understanding, abilities and capacity to change improves

5. Give your clients simple solutions to their most pressing issues and leave the rest till later

6. Don't be concerned with what other people and trainers think; do the best thing for the client at that point in time. The opinions of others are irrelevant

The title of this chapter might have led you to believe that I was going to tell you exactly how to assess a client. Sorry, but that's an impossible task to accomplish through a book. The art of assessing is a hands on skill which you should learn by doing and doing often. I want to address the communication aspects of your coach/client relationship which is so often overlooked and yet so vitally important in our roles as personal trainers.

If you would like to improve your knowledge of the assessment process, then I suggest you re-visit your course manuals or attend CPD workshops that can teach you the soft skills on movement assessment and delivering training to a client. If you want to build your nutrition knowledge, then consider enrolling on the The BTN Academy Academy: the nutrition course that I teach with other top experts from the industry.

Summary: The assessment process

- Listen to your client

- Every situation is different: context is key

- Keep things as simple as possible to implement for the client

- Be aware of your client's expectations from your initial working relationship

- Give your clients what they need and don't bombard them with unnecessary information

- Keep listening

- Develop trust and only advance your clients when they're ready

- Then, when the client is ready, challenge them with something that pushes them to show them what they are really capable of

CHAPTER 6
THE LOCK-IN

We're not down the pub, so don't get too excited. And we're fitness professionals, why would we be in the pub? After all, we don't drink...

All jokes aside, it's time to get serious on one of the most effective techniques I can give you for turning your business around.

We live in a tech-savvy society full of electronic gadgets and distractions. Look around you and I guarantee you won't have to look far to see someone glued to their phone screen. Perhaps you're guilty of this too.

As fitness professionals, this habit needs to change. But why?

Because it's stopping you from being more successful.

Don't get me wrong, I love social media: it's an incredible tool. But for many it's an addiction. Every spare second is spent on Facebook or Instagram looking at the latest updated feed or generally wasting time absorbing unnecessary information. That doesn't mean I'm against using social media to find new and interesting things to learn, as I've mentioned already, social media is a wonderful way to connect to others and be inspired. But there has to be a limit.

I decided to take action in my own life. And it's those actions that play a key role in improving my business model. When I get up in the morning, I don't turn on my phone. For me, 6-10am is my time. It's the most precious part of my day and you'd have to beg, borrow and steal to take that time away from me. It's also the time when I'm my most productive and do my best work, whether that be writing, developing programs, scheming or dreaming. I make use of that deep concentration and focus and get to work on the most important jobs that day. When I'm finished, only then do I turn on my phone.

Now most of you I imagine will be up at the crack of dawn to train your early morning clients. I understand that my routine would not be feasible for everyone's lifestyle. But the point I'm trying to make here is still relevant, regardless of when you dedicate time to yourself. If you want your business to flourish, you must dedicate the time to work ON your business, not IN your business.

Your own time starts by switching off your phone.

It's time to focus on you. You spend all day, all week and all month working in your business. What if I proposed that you take just one weekend off where you completely shut off from the world and worked ON your business. Away from social media and away from the distractions of the internet.

If you can't possibly imagine doing this, do you deserve to have a more successful business?

No, you don't.

Your business won't improve by accident. Developing your business starts with you. You need to take time for yourself to develop your ideas and ultimately create the action that drives your personal training business towards success.

Let's commit to a date now. Write down a date in which you will dedicate one whole weekend to working on your business. No family commitments, no clients, no appointments, no TV, no phone. Nothing. Don't worry, the world won't melt and Facebook will still be there when you re-start your week on Monday. Nothing will have changed, except your business. I guarantee you will start Monday morning with more enthusiasm and a re-ignited passion for your business, it's impossible not to.

There are two choices when it comes to developing your business. Continue as you are, slowly implementing the advice from this book (I hope), or smash a super productive weekend and turn your business on its head.

I do this all the time. I'm doing it right now writing this book.

I'm in lock-in mode: no phone, no appointments, nothing. It's just me and my writing, the occasional dog walk to keep my mind fresh, a workout in the afternoon in my garage gym (I don't leave the house to go to the gym, I like to stay close to home to keep my state of flow), good food to keep my brain energised and a quick 20 minute power nap when I need it. The result: I'm one motivated son of a gun.

Which I'll have written in 7 full days. 50,000 words in a week, who said it was hard work writing a book!

It's amazing what you can do in a short space of time when you put your mind to it and shut off the world.

So, write down your date.

Look ahead in your diary now and anticipate when you will have finished reading this book. Commit yourself to a weekend where you can go into lock-in mode and take your business up a notch.

The date of my lock in: _____

Sweet. Music to my ears. I love it when a plan comes together.

Once you've finished this book you should know everything that you must do, or should do, to improve your business. Then it's a case of planning your lock in, and doing it.

When it comes around, your lock-in plan might look like this:

1. Re-read the chapters you need a refresher on

2. Write down the key areas in your business that you need to improve on

3. Create strategies to implement change

4. Take the actions you need to improve those key areas e.g. contacting others, networking, purchasing items, get X app, send X emails

5. Be critical of your process: could your plans and actions be improved upon?

6. Ask someone else to critically review your plans and actions to highlight further improvements

7. Ensure all changes are implemented and let your family, business associates and clients know of any appropriate changes when relevant

Here's another little technique that I like to use in my own business. I suggest you purchase a white board from Amazon or get some large sheets of paper and plan topics for the date you committed to for your lock-in. Use your whiteboard (or paper) to brainstorm ideas and put it somewhere where you can see it daily. I prefer a whiteboard as I can make changes and continually add to my vision. Dedicating time to this lock-in process will have more of a positive effect on your business than ANYTHING. Trust me. I do it all the time and it shows in my success.

Commit to your lock-in date. Turn off your phone. Switch off from Facebook and plan: create a strategy and implement action.

And enjoy the fruits of more successful personal training business.

Speaking of your personal training business, let's talk customer service.

CHAPTER 7
CUSTOMER SERVICE

The term 'customer service' immediately conjures up the image of a retail environment and as personal trainers, we don't often think of ourselves as being in a customer service role. However, in a gym setting, good customer service is a fundamental aspect of any personal training business. Customer service in our industry is showing your clients that you genuinely care for their needs.

In Chapter 5 we discussed the assessment process and it is during this assessment process that your duty of care will grow. In fact, when we think about it, customer care really begins with the initial conversation you have when you first meet your prospective client.

It's the truth!

I recently surveyed the followers of my Facebook page which, at the time of writing, is almost 64,000 people. I wrote a post asking their opinions on character traits they dislike seeing in a personal trainer. Many of my followers felt that their personal trainer didn't care about them outside of their training hours. No additional support: just turn up, train, leave and we'll see each other again next week.

Do you think that's an example of good customer service?

Think back to the last time you were truly impressed by an item that you purchased. You probably already had an expectation of what it was going to be like to own it, but there were likely other factors that added to the experience that impressed you more than the product alone. Perhaps it was packaged in a nice box or it arrived pre-wrapped. The purchase may have been followed up with a phone call or the sales person went out of their way to find the right size for you. Giving awesome customer service isn't about giving what's expected, it's about giving the unexpected, that little bit more.

Think about the service you give to your clients. How would you rate your personal training service? And what does that service include? An hour's training session, maybe a text during the week to schedule the next session if the client is not already booked and the odd nutritional tip here and there.

If you received that service, would you be impressed?

I wouldn't. And I hope you wouldn't either. From your lock-in date and beyond you are going to give AWESOME customer service to your client. It all starts by showing them that you care.

My new client: The process

I want you to imagine that I'm now your personal trainer and we're about to embark on a journey together. Here's how our relationship pans out over the next 6-9 months…

You ring me up to book a trial session or a free consultation. During this phone call, I ask you for your email address to send over some details for you to look through before our training session begins.

After the phone call, I get on my laptop and send you an email containing confirmation of your appointment, directions on where to go and details on items to bring with you for your session. I may even give you a few tips on what to eat before training to ensure you have enough energy, plus any other relevant information gathered from our initial conversation.

At your first session, I'm waiting to greet you at reception or wherever I promised to meet you; I'm on time and exactly where we had planned to meet. I have a small hand towel with me that you can choose to use and a spare bottle of water in case you didn't bring one (whether you choose to use it or not, the gesture is still the same). During the session or consultation, I am attentive. I listen to you and we talk about you and your goals as much as possible.

We book you in for your next session that day. That evening (or the next day), I text you to let you know what a pleasure it was to meet you and that I'm looking forward to working with you over the coming months. I then send another pre-planned email with some useful information for our next session: what to expect, adding in a few relevant nutrition tips and mentioning that the next session might be a bit harder than the first one.

24 hours before your next session, I send you a reminder text for the session and use this contact as an opportunity for you to inform me of any issues I need to know about prior to our first proper session together.

I'm ready and waiting on time for you to start our next session. I've bought a nice colourful reusable water bottle for you (spending about £3-4) to keep in your gym bag. I've also presented you with a short 8-page nutrition booklet for you to read in your own time. We can discuss any nutritional queries in the last 10-15 minutes of your session. If not already booked, we set the date of our next session. I then send you a follow-up email reminding you to look over the nutrition booklet over the coming days and to come prepped with any questions for the next session. Session by session we'll address your nutritional concerns or questions that you may have.

We've now been training together for a few weeks and I've noticed you've been getting sore wrists; I buy you some wrist wraps (£5-7 off Amazon) and give them to you at your next training session. I want to ensure you're properly equipped and staying safe during your sessions with me.

The next week I send you a Whatsapp message with a link to an audio book on mind-set and food as I know this is something you've been struggling with after some recent chats.

Fast forward 6 weeks into your plan and I invite you to a Bootcamp training session with my other clients. The session is fun and informal and will cost you £5 instead of the normal £30. It's an opportunity for you to try a different style of training and to meet some like-minded people. There's the option afterwards to have lunch together at a new pub that does a nice range of healthy meals.

It just so happens that it's your birthday on the same week: I surprise you with a card and have gifted your next session free for your birthday.

A couple of months have passed and we're now into January. I'm starting a free Facebook group for all my clients that focuses on nutrition tips and recipes. I invite you to join as a way to stay accountable with your nutrition, learn some new recipes and have a place to ask for any nutrition advice.

As a special offer, I'm also having a 'Bring a Friend Week' where you will get 1/3 off your training if you bring a friend along to the session. I then extend my January training offer to your friend (who has now joined) who can bring her friend along for a session. There are now options for you to train with me in a semi-private session which works out cheaper per hour for you.

Side note: The more sessions you do that are semi-private or small group as opposed to 1-2-1s, the more you can earn. It's also an attractive option to a client. Let's imagine a client sees your pricelist as follows:

- 1-2-1 Training is £35 per hour
- Block of 10x 1-2-1 sessions is £300
- Semi-private training is £20 per hour
- Group training as a group of 12 is £5 per hour, see my class timetable for more info

I could then expand the above to include direct debits and other payment methods, but by training with others, your client will see the financial savings to be made. They can get the same service at a cheaper rate, your client is saving money and you're training more clients in less hours. Everyone wins.

I'm doing another Bootcamp this Saturday, £5 to participate with the option to go for a late breakfast afterwards at a local food shop that does some really nice protein pancakes loaded with fresh fruit.

Out of the blue, I drop you a Whatsapp voice memo on your phone and let you know about a new shop that sells paints for arts and crafts that has opened in town on Smithonian Street. I remember from our sessions together that you love arts and crafts in your spare time as your hobby and I thought you would like to know about the new shop.

We've been struggling with an area of your training for some time so I surprise you during today's session with one of the other trainers from the gym (I've asked him as a favour because I know it's his speciality subject). He's going to look at the problems and help us with a solution moving forward, two minds being better than one.

I'm hoping that if someone said to you now: "Oh I see you get personal training, what's your trainer like?" that you would say...

"My personal trainer is AWESOME!"

The scenarios I've just described above are a snapshot of my duties to you that show I truly care about you as a person and value you as my client. You're not just paying money for an hour of training at the gym, you're paying for someone to take real care in working with you to get your desired results.

Of course, I understand that not all the above suggestions will fit your environment. Be objective and think of ways in which you can apply those tips to your client's personal training sessions or think of some new ones on your own. None of this advice is new, it's all traditional customer service and it's time the fitness industry cared more about customer service. If we did, then people might have more good things to say about personal trainers.

For the general public, £30 is a lot of money to pay for an hour of personal training. Over deliver on your service and you can confidently justify your fee.

At the time of writing this book I charge £90 an hour, with this fee rising in the New Year. I always go above and beyond to deliver more to the client than they were expecting. Instead of them saying "My session with Ben was good", they say "My session with Ben was AWESOME, it absolutely blew my mind! I have so much more knowledge now to succeed and I feel really inspired".

That's customer service.

Implementing a system

The ideas I've listed in this chapter may seem like a lot of effort but the more you do them, the more habitual these practices become. Sending a client regular emails and reminder texts and buying them a water bottle only becomes an effort if you fail to organise your time effectively. It's up to you to plan for your success. Carrying out these simple gestures consistently is no different to reminding your client of the importance of sleep and hydration. Over time it becomes a habit. And it's a worthwhile task if you're serious about improving the quality of service to your clients.

If you look at your diary every day to see who you're training with, then this next task is no different. Sit down for 15-30 minutes each day and commit to your customer service duties for all of your clients. You may be sending an introductory email to one client and a follow-up email to another. Send a reminder text, buy a water bottle, prepare for the consultation with your new client and buy a birthday card for the client whose birthday's coming up next week.

You get the picture.

Make customer service a part of your daily routine. Create actions that show your clients you truly care and find things that work for you; don't do think because you feel you ought to. Show your clients you genuinely value them. If it's a forced act of kindness then it's not worth doing at all, and it will show.

The lock-in: Improving your customer service

Below is a checklist that you can use on your lock-in days to improve the customer service you provide for your clients:

1. Have a draft set of emails that you can personalise and send to clients at different stages of their journey and always remember to get the right name

2. Think of gifts for your clients that would benefit them on their fitness journey and source them in advance

3. Have pre-written documents to send to clients. Examples of ideas include a nutrition information booklet and hydration tip sheets. Prepare in advance, it takes a couple of minutes to send an email to your clients

4. Have an excel spreadsheet on all your clients and note their contact details, where they are on their journey, and any other relevant information that you can easily refer to as part of your daily customer service routine

The extra 15-30 mins of work that you commit to this task each day will produce noticeable differences in your business. Your word of mouth marketing is going to increase; your client's satisfaction will be huge and their results will prove that. You'll be providing your clients with a personal training experience like no other.

Not only are you providing a better service, you're providing yourself with a more efficient business. You're intelligently providing a gateway to upsell your clients into semi-private training, decreasing your working hours with no loss to the client. A smarter system and a better work life balance.

If you've yet to implement it, plan your lock-in date. And commit to having AWESOME customer service.

CHAPTER 8
ATHLETE STATUS

Many personal trainers aspire to have the support of a sponsorship. There's nothing more satisfying than the thought of working with a big company; you get to buy items at a discount and you might even get products for free. Everyone likes free stuff.

But before you involve yourself with a big brand, be wary of the company that you keep.

For the most part, running your personal training business on a day-to-day basis is your responsibility. You control your own content. The actions that a sponsored company makes, however, are out of your hands and those actions have the potential to taint your personal brand.

Now before we go any further, let's define the word 'brand': as a personal trainer, you are your own brand. You are responsible for the content you send out in your emails, for the pictures you post on your social media and for the image you portray a personal training professional.

A sponsored brand is no different. Their message, values, actions, online posts, training videos and sponsored athletes all combine to make up their brand. And should you choose to be associated with them, all those actions are subsequently linked to you. Sponsorship can enhance or detract from your own business success so it's important to choose wisely.

The company you keep is key.

An opportunity for sponsorship requires a serious consideration of your values. This can often be hard when there's financial pull for a short-term gain. But it's vitally important to consider the long-term effects of a sponsorship on your personal brand. Does the company in question carry out practices or sell items that could damage your brand long-term in ANY way if a client or associate saw it?

Let's imagine you've been approached by a supplement company. The following scenario is equally relatable to a clothing company, food snacks company, meal prep, diet shakes and so on. This supplement company has approached you and would love for you to be an ambassador for their brand. In exchange for your support, they will provide you with one of the following options:

1. Commission on people you refer to the brand (affiliate kick-back)
2. Discounted supplements and a commission for referrals
3. Free supplements and a commission for referrals
4. And if you're a really big deal, you might get paid a fee just for your association with the company

Sponsorship works in many ways but the idea is the same: at this point it seems as though you're benefitting from the relationship and are excited by the prospects of being affiliated with a bigger brand. Whether it's free stash or money, you're ready to jump in!

As you browse the company's website, you can imagine using 50% of their products; those products are items you would either use yourself or would recommend to clients. The other 50% are things you wouldn't use or necessarily agree with; it's irrelevant so you ignore them.

Let's say you're promoting a set of values to your clients that looks something like this:

1. Eat real food 80-90% of the time
2. Have a lifestyle that is low stress
3. Take part in training that you enjoy
4. Know when to push yourself and know when to scale your training back
5. Take supplements that are scientifically proven to be beneficial
6. Lose body fat by eating in a calorie deficit, not by resorting to a magic diet pill
7. Laugh lots and be fit to live a better life

Now those are just some examples which form part of my thoughts, opinions and values. I would hope that as whole, yours would be similar.

Now if your chosen supplement company only aligns with 50% of your values and you know they promote products or ideals that you wouldn't agree with, then this is a problem.

By association, you're potentially promoting values or products that go against your personal branding. In addition, you're introducing your clients to the company's social media channels. Clients are then exposed to conflicting information. Who can they trust?

For example: the company in question posts an Instagram post with one of their athletes promoting a low-carb diet to maximise fat loss. You don't agree with the advice that they've recommended and it's not the information you teach your clients. The next week there is a Facebook post about going hard or going home with a steroid-fuelled athlete proclaiming that their fat burners are the most effective method of fat-loss. You then find out from your clients that the company's recent monthly email pushed the fact that you NEED a recovery shake after training when you know that isn't true. You tell your client's it's optional, but it's not necessary. Your client sees you promoting this brand and questions why you're promoting something you don't believe in.

It all starts to get confusing and conflicted for the client, who is right?

The big brand with all the power and the athletes and shiny big promises, or my trainer?

Regardless of whether you choose to believe the company's messages, their opinions and marketing all link back to you. You may not agree with the messages being promoted or the lifestyle choices certain athletes make but you're now associated with that image. And now your clients are becoming influenced by this company's marketing. Those messages are now in direct conflict with you and what you are trying to teach them. And if your chosen company is promoting a quicker result over your advice, then you're fighting an uphill battle with your clients. You may be trying to teach them the truth surrounding diet, training and a healthy lifestyle, but if there's a quicker option that can be bought through their trainer's trusted brand then why bother with the long-winded lifestyle changes?

By association, you've chosen to support a company that you don't always agree with. You may only be supportive of 50% of their products and marketing but your clients are subjected to the entire ethos of the company. Their ideologies merge and whether you like it or not, become part of the package you sell within your personal brand.

You ignored the bits you didn't like because you were blinded by the shiny free stuff and the chance to be associated with a big brand.

In my own experience, I've been associated with companies in the past that put out products or statements that would have me shaking my head, questioning what's been said or cringing when I saw a new product that's being sold. And it always comes back to bite me. Nowadays I'm very picky with who I work with and haven't worked with a huge number of people in recent years because of this.

When working with, or recommending companies, it is essential that their ethos is in alignment with what you believe in and what you promote. This is one reason why I set up Awesome Supplements. I struggled to find a supplement brand that I resonated with that didn't sell bogus supplements like CLA and fat burners, and promoted values and ideals that I could be fully on board with.

You might look at Awesome Supplements and think: "I really believe in what they're doing. This is a brand I would happily recommend to my clients". If that's the case, please do sign up and join us in the fight to put better information out in the supplement world (which you can do by dropping by www.awesomesupplements.co.uk and applying for a trade, ambassador or affiliate account).

If you don't agree with Awesome Supplements, or any other brands that you are or could be associated with, don't associate yourself with them. You owe it to yourself to support your own brand or company with products you genuinely believe in. Your business is worth more than short-term commission or a discount card or some free protein.

There's nothing worse than having one of your clients enquire about something they have seen on Facebook that contradicts what you were talking about the week before. And it's even worse when it's posted by a company you recommend. Worse again is when you then have a client telling you that they bought products from an advert recommended by your sponsor company. You're totally against the products sold in the advert, but you're involved by association. And now your client is taking fat burners to help them improve their weight loss because of it.

This is NOT the client's fault, it's your fault. You chose to associate yourself with a sponsor company and their advertising. Clients are going to find this stuff online as soon as they start snooping around your Instagram profile or other social media posts.

Choose wisely. Select brands and products that you genuinely believe in and resonate with. Don't get lured in with a few free supplements or a new vest, think of the bigger picture. Your personal brand is far too valuable and you don't need the repercussions of a bad choice further down the line.

Do your research and hunt down all the companies you like and support and ask to join their ambassador programs. If a company doesn't have one because they are new, enquire all the same. You will likely be the impetus for them to create one; find the companies that sit with your values and ideals and align with them, not with companies that don't.

Don't get blinded by shiny free stuff, your brand is worth more than that.

And the same goes with sharing stuff online. Ensure that the videos, posts, pictures and memes that you share online are of people and companies that you resonate and agree with 99% of the time. If there is the odd post that you see and think "that's awesome, I'll share that", think twice and see if it is from a company or person you usually don't agree with. If so don't share it, because you run the risk of a client following that person or company and then they're being exposed most of the time to the wrong stuff.

It's all got to add up to 80-90% good, if not more, otherwise the little bits of bad or things you disagree with will come back to haunt you and you'll be performing damage limitation afterwards.

Think long-term. Poor decisions and short-term gains will always come back to bite you.

CHAPTER 9
ARE OTHER PERSONAL
TRAINERS YOUR COMPETITION ?

When I look back on my days at Fitness First in Hull (RIP), the atmosphere was fierce. Competition between personal trainers was high and we were all striving to be the best. Sure, I was nice to everyone and I had a lot of good friends that I worked alongside. But when it came to business, we were enemies. If I saw another personal trainer talking to a prospective client, my mind would go into overdrive: "How can I show that gym member that I'm the better trainer? He should be training with me. Can I approach him afterwards without that other trainer knowing?"

It's a dangerous thought process and sadly not uncommon in the commercial gym environment. This competitive nature breeds a culture that allows personal trainers to be guilty of the following traits:

- Arrogance towards members and other trainers
- Always proving their worth to everyone around them
- Territorial behaviour on the gym floor
- Talking negatively about other trainers in an effort to gain new clients
- Using tactical marketing that puts other trainers down
- Being unsupportive of other trainers in meetings with management, purely for personal gain
- Undercutting pricing to make more sales
- Offering deals to beat another trainer's deals
- Copying other trainers to appear more knowledgeable, in an attempt to justify their own ego

Let's be objective for a moment. Having listed those character traits, are you guilty of any of them?

Honestly.

I was guilty of many of those traits and having reflected on my past mistakes, I'm appalled by myself.

Think about the theme running throughout this book. Most of the admirable traits of a personal trainer come from being a good human being. Do the qualities above reflect the actions of a good human being? Do they show kindness, support and indicate the game plan for success?

No. Not in the slightest. The only outcome this behaviour breeds is contempt and dislike and those same character traits will be used against you too. If you create this environment in your gym and a new trainer arrives, they will begin to adopt the same traits as you. In time they will become a product of their environment, an environment that YOU have influenced. An environment that breeds unhealthy competition, back-stabbing and an embarrassing display of ego. And ultimately your behaviour has a negative effect on the most important person that we've yet to mention in this chapter...

...the client.

We're thinking about ourselves, again. What can WE gain from the situation. It's no longer about the client and who we can help, it all boils down to what we can gain financially from the failure of others.

Let me propose a paradigm shift that I think the fitness industry badly needs and that should be adopted in every gym in the world. But first...

Context

I'm fortunate to know a lot of successful gym owners who own a variety of small, medium, large, and often multiple gym facilities. The success within any of those gyms is largely dependent on a solid team of staff who work well together. Everyone works as a unit, supporting one another and helping one another out. They don't breed competitive behaviour; the team builds success together.

Can you name a successful company that has been built, long term, on negativity, back-stabbing and a failure to work as a unit? Not likely.

I understand that within many gym environments a personal trainer is working in a self-employed role. And a large portion of that role requires you to build your income to support your lifestyle and pay your bills. But whether you realise it or not, you are part of a team. Choose to focus on your own greed and you're bound to fail.

How do I know this? Because I failed at that Fitness First gym in Hull. I only ever had 4-5 clients at any given time, even after 2 years of being there.

I've learnt, reflected and applied.

Let's fast forward for some more context

After finishing university in June 2010, I hung around for 6 months working in Hull with my many jobs (I worked as a kids rugby coach 6-12 hours a week, worked shifts in a cocktail bar 3 nights a week, had 2 shifts a week in a local off-licence and all while trying to build and grow The BTN Academy (BTN). I then made plans to travel over to Dubai and Abu Dhabi (UAE) for December for a month to scope out opportunities for my future. I was working hard: trying, failing, and learning with every new experience.

(I know, I'm a hustler: It's called hard work. Good things happen when you work hard).

Top Tip: if you're still trying to work out what to do, or are wanting more time to learn and shape your craft, get a job that enables you to study while you earn money. I worked in an off-licence part time; when the shop was quiet I would study, write blogs for BTN, and research things I was learning or doing. When I was 18 I also had a van drivers job and a bar job where I did the same. As long as I was doing my job, I would find any opportunity to learn at the same time. It helps you build your future while taking care of the all-important finances. That doesn't mean not doing your job, that's disrespectful to your employer and to the pay you're receiving. Do your job, but use your time wisely to earn while you learn. I did, and look where that got me!

UAE

I headed out to the UAE to explore Dubai and Abu Dhabi for its potential opportunities and a much-needed break away from the grind. During my month break I had A LOT of time to think. I had the time to enjoy living, eating, playing, exploring and building BTN part time. More importantly, it gave me the time to explore the ideas going around in my head as a young man post uni with his career ahead of him (age 24).

It was a combination of this time alone reflecting and going for interviews in gyms in the UAE that I started to piece together how to be an AWESOME coach. Now don't get me wrong, there are many 'moments' of which I am explaining and exploring in this book that pieced together the skills of a great personal trainer, but this particular example is directly associated to this chapter.

I started to reflect on why I wasn't a successful trainer at Fitness First. Why couldn't I get clients? Why was Tom more successful than me? Why after 2 years in that gym was I still struggling on 4-5 clients a week and surviving on my paid gym instructor time and my other jobs?

I applied and attended 12 interviews during that month in the UAE and my experiences gave me the impression that the commercial gym environment was a horrible place work in. Up until this point I'd only ever worked in 2 gyms, the private facility I started in before I went to university (ReFresh Fitnesss in Ipswich) and Fitness First at university. As a gym user I'd only ever been in two other gyms; a David Lloyd in Ipswich when I was on my weight loss journey and my university student gym. The experience of those 12 interviews gave me a feel for what was really happening in the wider gym environment: how they operated, what the staff were like, what the members were doing, the culture the managers set and the energy of the overall environment.

It was essential to get a feel for the place I might be working in, so after every interview I would do a workout in the gym. During my training sessions at those gyms I would be receptive to my environment, observing the other trainers and their behaviour. I would also, where possible, try and chat with the trainers as a customer. Then I'd drop in the line that I was thinking of taking a job there.

9 times out of 10, guess what happened?

They became short and defensive. They changed their posture, gave short answers to my questions and soon found an excuse to move on from the conversation. It gave off an uninspiring and unsupportive message and it just didn't feel right. I had come to loathe the behaviour the gym bred and how that had influenced my training methods.

That list of all the negative character traits I wrote at the beginning of this chapter was apparent in those gyms I visited. Why was this the norm?

This needed to change.

Or to be more specific, I needed to be the change.

And this is what I am going to ask of you now: be the change the fitness industry needs.

My 2nd commercial gym job, David Lloyd Ipswich

After being in the UAE for a month, I knew it wasn't the place for me. Still questioning my abilities to make BTN a success and with no set career path, I decided to apply for a job with the RAF. My dad is in the military and convinced me it was a solid career path; there were training roles (PTI) within the RAF that I would be capable of, but deep down I knew it would never make me happy. I explored the option regardless and applied to be a RAF PTI and decided to head back home, moving back in to my parents house that was rented out to various people living in the rooms. It wasn't the environment I wanted to be in, but it was the best I had and it was free rent while I got myself on my feet.

I was hoping my new drive to make something of myself would impact on my personal training skills on the gym floor.

So, the life plan at this stage, January 2011, was as follows: go home, work as a personal trainer 30-40 hours per week, train for my RAF test, and grow BTN: blog, make videos, coach clients online, and make it work, I believed in it and wanted to make it work.

On arriving home, I started training immediately for my RAF test having been accepted via my initial application. I also applied for a new job in the original David Lloyd gym I had joined on my weight loss journey. Thankfully I got the position and having reflected on my previous mistakes as a personal trainer after my time away in the UAE I was insistent on making a success of this job, and of myself.

I decided from that day on that this would be my personal training manifesto:

- Be kind and supportive to every trainer in the gym
- Act with ZERO ego, both to members and the other trainers
- Genuinely seek opportunities to help clients with free advice and be the go-to guy
- Avoid wearing tight t-shirts around the gym to prove myself
- To clean the equipment and carry out all aspects of my job with pride
- To recommend other trainers in the gym when I know they can do a better job than me with a client due to their specialities
- To act as the linchpin of the training team and always strive to bring people together
- Be kind and supportive to all the gym members
- Be likeable, be the guy that people wanted to be around

My actions reflected positively all around me and I really loved my job as a result of this. A lot. Being honest, this was the first time that deep down I enjoyed being a personal trainer. I had more job satisfaction, I was liked, there was a team ethos, we had fun and there was no bitching between staff. I went in and came out every day smiling.

And guess what?

I had enough clients to support myself within 7 weeks. Now I was fully booked with training sessions. My efforts were paying off.

Now I didn't stay at that gym much longer as I got offered another opportunity. I could happily have stayed there and built my business to an even larger status, but the opportunity was too good to pass up.

My short time at this gym doesn't change what happened with my experience and how quickly I built up my business. That still stands. These lessons still stand. What you learn from this still stands. Just because things changed for me so quickly it doesn't take away from what success I had when I changed my personal training manifesto.

But, the grass got greener very quickly for me, so I walked on it.

The rugby club

When I arrived home I went back to my old rugby club and started to take up the sport again. After a couple of weeks, the club manager asked what I was doing with myself now I was back (at this point I'd been away from the club for almost 4 years) and I explained my current situation: personal trainer at David Lloyd gym by day, working on building BTN by night. He then asked if I would run strength and conditioning based sessions for the team; the lads needed extra sessions to work on their match fitness and the current coach wasn't available during the week to do more than he was currently doing.

At first, I politely declined. Between working my personal training shifts, the unpredictability of my clients and working on BTN, I was too busy. He then suggested using the club's gym to train my clients, for free, in exchange for training the team. During the day the club was barely in use and I could come and go as I pleased, I wouldn't have to do my 20 hours at the gym and that free time could be better spent training clients and doing something I love.

For me it was silly not to take the deal and I can imagine if you were in my shoes you would have too. I loved helping the rugby club and I loved training my clients; giving up 2 hours a week for free use of a well-equipped gym was a no brainer. I was in. My only concern was my clients: would they continue to train with me if I moved elsewhere?

Thankfully when I discussed the changes, 6 of my 7 clients chose to follow me to the rugby club. It was a better working environment for me and there was more flexibility and options to train for them. A win-win situation all round. I handed in my resignation to David Lloyd, they understood my reasons and wished me well.

So here I am, now training clients at the rugby club 15-20 hours a week, helping the boys at the club and dedicating the rest of my time to working on BTN.

I had found my path, life was good.

And for the record, I failed my RAF test before I even got to it. I received the letter after several months of training, informing me that under 2nd phase review of my application, I was a security risk as I had travelled so much in the past. My previous backpacking trips to Asia, Europe and Central America and my stint in the Middle East deemed me a security threat, and so my application was void. Weird, but hey, such is life, it just proved the path I was on was the right one.

My personal training career then flourished being self-employed working out of the gym. I had another good year of personal training before BTN then demanded more of my time, eventually allowing me to leave my life as a personal trainer in exchange for full-time coaching online. But that's a story for another chapter.

Fate eventually showed its path, it always does.

The paradigm shift

What kind personal trainer are you going to choose to be?

I hope you're choosing to be the latter; to be the personal trainer that is kind, supportive and a team player. To lay your ego aside and think of the interests of your clients. To support your fellow trainers rather than compete against them.

Don't choose to follow the crowd and blame your negative qualities on the attitudes and actions of other trainers. It's an embarrassing excuse. Choose to be responsible for your own actions and a better person. It can be difficult when others around you are competitive, disingenuous, and unsupportive of one another.

Be the change.

I want you to be different. This book is about you being AWESOME, not staying the same as every other trainer. Be the change you want to see in the industry and others will follow.

Strategies to create change

So how do you change your gym's environment? The way I see it, there are 3 methods of attack:

First: Change begins with you. You can choose to be supportive, kind, genuine and humble to your team. Share knowledge, learn from one another and refer clients to other trainers who have a better speciality for their needs. Your actions and genuine intentions are the foundations for creating a better team environment. Your behaviour will start to rub off on other people; they will see that you're creating a better way of doing things and slowly they'll come to realise that a more positive working environment is beneficial to everyone in the gym.

Second: Speak to management and inform them of your observations regarding the team environment. Let them know that you'd like to work together with them to improve the team's ethos and to build a better way of working as a unit. Request a team meeting to discuss strategies to improve the working relations of the team. Organising a social event is one way to get to know each other outside of the gym and to improve communication. You might even recommend this book to the other trainers, or to management and suggest they recommend the team read it.

Third: If management don't support your ideas for change then get the phone numbers of all the trainers at the gym and create a WhatsApp or social media group. Arrange an available date to organise your own team meeting. Explain that that you have some great ideas that everyone will benefit from and that the meeting will address ways to collectively get more clients, work more effectively together, help one another, create a referral system and generate greater job satisfaction.

If you are willing to believe your actions will work, they will.

If you don't believe it can work, it won't. People will see that your intentions are not genuine and the change will be lacklustre. They may feel you're only trying to create change to better your own position within the gym which is only going to create further hostility and no real change. Be clear on your intentions, approach this activity with a confidence and genuine passion to make change happen.

Photocopy this chapter (or take photos on your phone; photocopiers are so 2005) and give it to every one of your team in the gym. Let them know that you wish to take action and organise a team meeting to get ideas flowing. Having read the chapter, they will have a better background understanding of why you're doing this and by getting involved themselves can work with you to create a change for the better.

Do it.

I promise your gym will be more pleasant to work in. You'll have greater job satisfaction, attract more clients, retain more of your existing clients and spend more time being a successful trainer. The average duration of a personal trainer's career is currently 12-18 months. That's a dire statistic that we need to change; this industry needs more passionate personal trainers working longer careers if it's going to change the state of the nation's health.

If there are 1 or 2 trainers who don't buy into your ideas, don't worry about it. You can't help everyone and it's unlikely that everyone will be supportive of your ideas in the beginning. If the majority of the team are willing to create this new team environment, the naysayers will come around in time when they see that change is working.

An important note...

If someone decides to change their mind and become involved in your teamwork, don't belittle them to prove your superiority. Welcome them with open arms and leave your ego at the door. Nothing is achieved with you trying to prove you are right.

If you're reading this book as a manager of a gym and have a team, please do this with your staff. Create a culture within your team that allows for passion and real job satisfaction. As I've previously mentioned, no truly successful team is ever built with insincere and hostile behaviour.

Final thoughts

There are enough clients in the world for every trainer to thrive and have a successful business. Don't be afraid to be honest and refer a client to someone else if there's a more suitable trainer for their needs. When I worked in David Lloyd, I referred a good handful of clients to other people. We had various trainers specialising in different aspects of training. Perhaps you can relate to the following trainers in your gym too:

Trainer 1 – Male competitive body builder. Specialised in training and nutrition for optimal body composition.

Trainer 2 – Female competitive body builder. Specialised in training and nutrition for optimal body composition.

Trainer 3 – Specialised in women over 30, often pre and post-natal clients looking for inspiration and changes in current lifestyle habits.

Trainer 4 – Specialised in group training, running outdoor bootcamps in the early morning and late evenings. Attracted clients who didn't want to pay for 1-2-1 sessions.

Trainer 5 – The all-rounder. Worked with male and female clients and specialised in improving their general health and fitness.

Trainer 6 – Me. Worked with younger male and female clients to improve posture, body composition and sporting performance. Specialised in sports players with health-related complaints.

I referred a number of people on to the bodybuilding trainers as I knew this was an area of expertise in which they would do a far better job than me. There was another instance when I had an older lady who I felt, given her background and goals, would be better placed with Trainer 3. Of course, this doesn't mean that I referred everyone away, but I owe it to the client to give them the best possible chance of success. And if someone else is better suited to empower them and get them to their goals quicker, then the client deserves to be referred on.

After doing this a couple of times, other trainers then started to refer people back to me. I became the go-to trainer for gut and stress-related issues; we referred clients out of respect for our team's skillset and ultimately the client would be the one to benefit.

This was team work.

Do you want to create the environment I created in that gym in a short space of time?

It starts by working as a team. As cliché as the phrase 'team work makes the dream work' sounds, it really is true. If you want the dream of the successful personal training business and genuine job satisfaction, work as a team not as a solo mercenary.

Other trainers aren't your competition, they are your friends, your colleagues, your peers and your team. Respect them.

CHAPTER 10
KISS YOUR CLIENTS

Don't kiss your clients, let's just put that one to bed straight away.

Shoot, another bad pun!

What does 'KISS' mean?

Keep It Simple, Stupid.

As a young and inexperienced trainer, I was skilled in the art of complicating everything. Crazy training programs, complex diets, unnecessary carb cycling, awkward stretches, I had it nailed. And while this stuff might have been useful to some clients, was it really all necessary?

Now some of this stuff might have been super useful to these clients, but were they ready for it? Could they mentally handle all this change? Think about your life when something changes? How do you respond? Do you always have the capacity to change multiple things at once? Or do you get overwhelmed?

There is a reason research indicates that slow and gradual habit change so that you can engrain it into your lifestyle is the most beneficial way to change, long term. Yet how many of you as coaches are asking their client to change their training, change their diet, change their lifestyle, change the way they think, just change EVERYTHING, right from the gate?

We've already covered some of these points in a roundabout way in the previous chapters, but I want to ensure that you understand the importance of Keeping It Simple. Remember the example with myself and Tom: Tom was the master of keeping things simple, taking his time and adding layers when the client was ready for change. Tom's clients trusted his methods and his techniques. I, on the other hand, bulldozed my way into my clients' lives and proclaimed that everything to be changed at once. And my success rate was low, 30-40% on average. Those are poor stats. And it wasn't that my clients were not ready to change, they were. They just weren't ready to be slapped in the face and shown how crap their life was all at once. They weren't ready to follow my perfect lifestyle and change everything immediately. It wasn't the best way to approach the situation.

Creating an all-or-nothing approach is likely to create 1 of 3 emotions or key character traits that we'll likely experience when training our clients:

1. **Elation** – The client is inspired, prepared and ready for change; client goes off and implements everything that you've asked them to

2. **Resistance** – The client is not open to being told everything in their life is wrong; they retaliate by closing up, resisting and make no changes

3. **Overwhelm** – Information overload becomes too much to process. No changes are made in this client

Here we can see the reasons why I only got 30-40% of people changing their habits with my approach; there is no single model of change that works for everyone.

So how do we approach each reaction type?

We can go full bore with Reaction 1 (elation) and use my approach. This client is receptive to lots of new information and are already in a high state of readiness to change. They're elated with the diet and training plan and just need the tools to do it. Let's go they say!

Reaction 2 resistance, on the other hand is apprehensive to change. In this situation, your approach needs to be based on education. Resistance can be caused by a number of factors: perhaps your client has a rigid set of beliefs that makes them eat a certain way, or would have them believe certain macronutrients are 'bad' for them. Their views may have caused them to become dogmatic in their opinions. We need time for them to warm to our views and ideas by giving them appropriate tools and resources that they can learn from.

Now in this scenario a small percentage of your education can come from a direct source, i.e. your client believes that carbs are bad and have a negative impact on weight loss, so you send your client an article on the science of carbohydrates and their role in caloric intake. Depending on their level of resistance, this may not be the best way to educate them early on, especially if challenging their belief system is likely to cause further resistance. A gentler, more passive form of teaching may be required.

The first step of passive coaching is simply to engage: talk to your client, train together and build rapport. Over time, the client develops a trust in you and is more receptive to your ideas. You've developed a relationship with them that they value; they now trust that your solutions to their problems may be better than their current belief structure.

The second step of coaching passively is to refer to a resource that you know and trust, allowing the client to tap into new knowledge on their own and build new beliefs and views over time. Instead of sending them an article on carbs being good, recommend a podcast that discusses the function of carbs and why we need them within our diet.

Here I'll use my podcast, Ben Coomber Radio as an example.

In Podcast Episode 117, I talk about building a diet from the ground up. Throughout the podcast, we discuss all aspects of diet and why each macronutrient is important. I'm not directly solving the problem yet, but I'm passively talking about all 3 of the macronutrients and their benefits. A few podcast episodes down the line, when the client has bought into the podcast and is enjoying the information, the show moves onto a question regarding carbohydrates and the importance of quantifying them in your diet, essentially, giving the listener all the facts.

Each podcast gives the client an opportunity to build on their knowledge. By listening to the podcasts, your client isn't feeling forced into changing their opinions. You'd be surprised how successful this form of learning can be. Five episodes later, your client is likely to be coming to their session talking about carbs in a totally different way: "Ben said on this week's podcast that carbs are ok, as long as I control my overall calorie intake and optimise the volume based on my training and how they make me feel. I've started eating more carbs after training and I feel as though I'm recovering better already and have more energy".

And there you have it, a simple two-step passive approach for dealing with resistance. Don't rush your horse to water: educate them and in their own time they'll drink.

What about Reaction 3, overwhelm?

Change in Character 3 is more emotionally challenging, they don't necessarily have resistance to knowledge, rather, they're stuck because they either don't believe in themselves, don't value themselves enough, lack self-confidence, or feel beaten down by their environment. Anything that adds an emotional challenge overwhelms them and they struggle to cope with the situation.

The best approach with this client is to give them exactly what they came to you for. Start training immediately, get them moving and allow them to see they're making positive changes from day 1. More importantly, be their friend. Start to understand them. Understand their emotions, the way they think and their problems: get on their level. For this client, you ideally want their training sessions to act as periods of respite, allowing them the opportunity to feel less overwhelmed and thus more empowered to make small changes when they have the mental capacity to do so.

It's all about peeling back the layers: using communication to contextualise the emotions and the problems they carry around with them daily and help, when possible, to overcome them. You can then begin to add the positive lifestyle changes back in when there's more mental and emotional clarity and willingness to embrace change.

Over time, as this client becomes stronger and more empowered, they'll be receptive to new learning opportunities. At this stage, DO NOT pile all your information onto them. At best it'll work for a few weeks, then something will happen in their lifestyle that takes them off-track. All of a sudden, everything you've asked them to do becomes too much. They skip a few training sessions, ditch the diet and slowly the emotional attachment to food begins to rear its head. That positive upward trajectory is now in a quick downward spiral, all because you asked too much of them as they juggled with their emotional issues, despite initially seeming ok.

Continue to go slow with this client.

They might think they're ready for more but hold strong and continue to layer things slowly. This character trait is too high risk to go fast unless you feel, by some divine intervention, that there's been a turnaround in their way of thinking. This can sometimes happen when a client leaves a partner that wasn't right for them, or leaves a job they disliked. In such instances, proceed quicker, but still proceed with caution. We don't want to cause a relapse.

As we've discussed in previous chapters, we need to exercise KISS with all our clients. We need to exercise it as an individual trainer and as an industry. We've made fitness and nutrition so unnecessarily complicated.

We need to simplify.

Take a look at some of your training plans, diet plans and recommendations that you give to your clients. Are they overly complicated? Are you asking too much of them? And what is your advice teaching them?

Are you teaching them to become independent? Or have you made fitness, nutrition and health seem so complicated that they always need a trainer or a programme to make progress and 'stay on track'?

If you look back on fitness from the 80s and 90s, people would exercise in a way that was fun, often in groups and classes, or simply by running or playing. They would eat a low fat diet of whole foods, drink lots of water where possible and that was it.

I'm not saying that was perfect, but it was simple. And for many it worked.

Maybe it worked because it was so simple and everyone could do it. I think there's a happy medium between those two examples, what we're doing now and what we might have done 20-30 years ago. That's for you to decide. You're the trainer, I'm just leading you to the water...

As I summarise this chapter, I want you to think about the way you're training your clients. Could you vary your approach to different character types and care for them in a way that makes them respond better? Could you keep your methods so simple that it's do-able for every client?

Because there's nothing wrong with a squat, some lunges, and a 20-minute run followed by an omelette and some fruit.

KISS.

CHAPTER 11
BELIEVE IN YOURSELF

Many trainers feel that they don't know enough to help their clients.

You look up to people that are more experienced in the industry, perhaps someone like me, or to other coaches and educators and think: "Ben Coomber knows X, Y and Z. I need to reach that level before I start talking about all this nutrition and training stuff".

But why are you comparing yourself to me? Or others that are perceived to be 'above' you?

Think about your job and what you aim to do; who are you aiming to help and attract to your services?

99% of the time you're aiming to help everyday people improve their health, body composition, performance, recovery and mindset. Your services will empower these people with the knowledge and the resources to help them reach their goals in the quickest way possible.

That's a completely different role to the one that I play in the fitness industry. My job is to train the everyday person just like you, but also to educate personal trainers and teach them to maximise their skills when working with clients. As I'm putting myself in a positon to educate and empower trainers, I should have the skills and knowledge to deliver on that, I should know more.

Why are you panicking when our roles are different?

I mentor a lot of trainers and am often asked for ways to improve on various aspects of their businesses. One area that frequently causes fear is the marketing of online services, or a coach's services in general. Many trainers are afraid of putting themselves 'out there' for fear of getting called out by other trainers or for fear of rejection at the hands of others opinions.

In other words, people are scared to look stupid.

With no disrespect to you, I'm not following your social media, and nor will others above you that you follow or look to for knowledge and guidance. I might see a post or 2 every now and again, but just like you, I'm looking through social media for information that can help me (so I'm looking 'above' too), or I'm connecting with friends and colleagues (looking side ways).

Do not fear what I will think of your marketing or the messages you are putting out there, I'm not looking at them, but, your clients are, so again let's think of your clients, and disregard your peers or the people above.

The process of knowledge acquisition (a key reason we are all on social media) follows a chain and I reckon that 99% of the time people are either looking up or looking side-to-side: we need to look down more, or more specifically, you need to look down more.

When looking side-to-side you see what your peers are doing. You engage with them and try to match their efforts. When looking up, you seek guidance, knowledge and advice. You might be looking up to my work for guidance towards greater success or increased knowledge; perhaps that's one of the key reasons why you chose to buy this book. But your marketing efforts online should be about the people below you and how you can serve them.

To set the record straight here, I don't regard myself as being higher up than you or better than you in any way. I bet that many of you reading this book have far more knowledge than I do and are actually better trainers than me.

But I am good at:

- Observing
- Explaining
- Simplifying
- Communicating
- Empowering
- Speaking
- Leading and helping others
- Creative thinking
- Problem solving
- Developing products people want and need

With those skills in mind, that's why I do what I do. That's why I branched out from personal training into mentoring and consulting and running a bigger fitness business, and chose to be a leader to the people in my company and to others that might want to learn from me.

If I'm not following you online and your aim is to inspire, market to, and convert everyday clients into your business, then why are you worried about what people like me are going to think when you post something online?

I'm not watching, or listening, but your clients are...

Your clients don't know what you know

It's important to remember that your clients only know a fraction of your knowledge. The valuable stuff that you should be talking about to others, people below you, should reflect that and be super simple. Let them know the importance of protein, fruit and vegetable intake, and all the foundational elements they need and should know. Guide them as you tackle the broscience in fitness and nutrition and reinforce the importance of hydration, sleep, recovery, finding enjoyment in training and the benefits of working out.

These things are so simple to you and me, but your clients don't know this stuff, or are struggling to implement it. Thus, you should and could be talking about this stuff all the time, on and offline. And you shouldn't worry about what others are thinking of what you are saying or posting.

How can you really screw up talking about protein to someone, or hydration, or training systems?

This stuff is simple, but it's important for everyone, especially your potential clients, the people below. No one is going to argue with you if you're outlining a few key facts about protein and why it's essential in the diet, so don't fear putting yourself out there and saying it, especially when your clients often struggle with the most basic of nutrition information.

You know enough to help your clients. Your Facebook posts, your marketing, your explanations to clients in a consultation don't need to be as complicated as my blogs or explanations. My target audience isn't your target audience. I need to be more technical, you don't.

Please don't think you don't know enough to help your clients, you likely do.

If you genuinely don't have enough knowledge because you haven't done a nutrition course yet, or you haven't yet completed your personal training course, then by all means your assumptions may be correct. But if you're reading this having completed a nutrition course like our The BTN Academy Academy, or your Personal Training level 3 course, you know enough to help 99% of people in your gym or online.

Your primary job is to reinforce the basics, it's what everyone needs. And more importantly, it's what your clients need.

The key aim of this chapter is to empower you and assure you that you are capable and knowledgeable enough to help people. Don't put yourself down. We often come into trouble or conflict when we're outside our comfort zones discussing subjects we're not comfortable with.

For example, if I was going to speak online about the Krebs Cycle (the APT energy cycle for sports performance and fuel utilisation), I would do my best to keep it simple, applicable and practical, just like we do in our nutrition courses. Going in-depth won't help more people and its often useless knowledge that's rarely used in a practical sense.

If I'm being honest, even I don't know all the inner workings to a deep scientific level about the Krebs cycle.

Why?

It doesn't and didn't help me do my job any better. When I did know it in detail back in the earlier days of my nutrition and fitness training (especially when I was studying for my CISSN) it didn't help me do my job better, so I stopped panicking that I needed to know it and focused on the info that actually helped people, boiling it all down into the 'need to know stuff'.

Thus, I wouldn't post about something of that nature in depth, because it wouldn't be true to me and what I teach, and I would be outside my comfort zone (which might lead me to panic or worry what others might think, because I have put myself in a compromised positon). If you never put yourself in that positon you don't ever give yourself an opportunity to fail. You can't get called out because there are no inconsistencies in what you are posting, everything is legit, and you only give yourself an opportunity to succeed.

And I want you to succeed.

You should want to succeed, every day.

That doesn't mean I don't value opportunities to learn, I love striving to be better. Every day I try and improve myself: my knowledge, what I do, and who I can help. But this NEVER stops me helping people with what I already know. Knowledge is a limitless thing. You will always be learning and you SHOULD always be learning.

So, where is the tipping point? When do you know enough to help others?

Like I said before, I never assume I'm the cleverest guy in the room or the most intelligent nutritionist. However, by the skill of being a good communicator, I'm confident that I can help 99% of people. I fully admit and appreciate that I'm not the best. And that's ok: it doesn't matter. I know enough to help you, so I do. You likely know enough to help your clients and the people that follow your work, so be confident and show that.

Don't ever think otherwise. Go out there and help your clients. Shout your knowledge from the rooftops.

And another thing: just because something has been said before doesn't mean it shouldn't be said again. So many trainers shy away from doing things because others have done them previously.

So what?

When I wrote my first blog on protein, do you think I was the only person to have ever written about the subject? Of course not. There are 1000s of people before me who have, but that doesn't matter. I'm not trying to service the people that have previously read someone else's account of protein intake, I'm talking to the people who follow my work.

I'm giving my account of protein; I want my opinion heard. And so should you.

Don't avoid doing things just because others have done so in the past. All this health and fitness knowledge needs to be repeated and told to as many people as possible. It's unlikely that your clients or followers follow me, and if they do, that's partly due to your influence and recommendations (thank you). Your clients, or potential clients, may never have read a blog about protein: serve to educate them. Share YOUR message, thoughts and ideas with the world and your clients.

Help the people below, don't look to appease people that are above, or sideways.

Don't hold yourself back: be assured that you're intelligent enough and know enough to help 99% of people who approach you for your services. Of course that doesn't mean avoid learning new skills or taking courses, always strive to better yourself. But be assured that you know enough to help your average client.

Believe in yourself.

You know enough, share it with the world and bring people up.

Don't fear the work of people above you, they're not looking down, but your clients are looking up, and that gives you the opportunity to help them.

It's your job to help them, share your message, thoughts and opinions.

CHAPTER 12
DELETE INSTAGRAM

Are you crazy Ben? Instagram is life!

Side note: I haven't considered the longevity of this book and fully expect some of you to read this in the future and ask yourself: 'WTF is Instagram?'. Should Instagram inexplicably disappear, it's a photo based social media platform that allows users to share clips of their life to others. It's a way to market your personal brand and share ideas, selfies and life experiences.

Further side note: I really hope Instagram doesn't disappear, I like it! And so should you. In my opinion it's one of the better social media platforms we have access to.

With the explosion of the online world, there is a pressure to be seen and heard online.

I don't want to burst your bubble but it could be the biggest waste of your time, EVER.

EVER, EVER, EVER, EVER, EVER.

Why?

Let me explain...

The online world is crowded and almost everyone we know is online. But generating a client-trainer relationship isn't as easy as putting up a few pictures and hoping you've persuaded people to buy into your services, far from it. Without personal interaction, there is no development of trust. Trust is vital to reassure potential clients that you can help deliver them the results they're looking for. And without trust, there is less willingness to buy into your training services.

So how do you build trust quickly and gain new clients?

By going out there and interacting.

We're often quick to judge our clients and complain that they're looking for the easy way out. They're the ones wanting to follow the extreme diet plan, take diet pills or drink shakes to lose weight. But replace the concept of weight loss with marketing and you may be just as guilty with your business model. That's one reason people resort to online marketing as a personal trainer: in principal, its easy.

In reality, it's not easy to become successful online. It took me 3 years before I developed any form of online success with my personal brand and Body Type Nutrition, and another 3 years of building on that to get to where we are today. That's 6 years of weekly blogs, posting ideas online, sharing recipes, filming videos and 4 years of a weekly podcast. All of these actions take up a massive amount of my time and effort. Marketing your brand online is far more challenging than marketing in a gym.

Anyways, enough of my journey and the online world, let's talk about you: what can you do to attract more clients?

If you want something in life, then take action to make it happen; get out of your comfort zone and interact with others. Let's look at 10 simple strategies you can use to attract more clients and make others aware of your business:

1. Talk to gym users on the gym floor: be humble, personable and likeable. Don't use this interaction as a sales pitch. Be genuine and look for opportunities to help. You want to build up a relationship whereby you're trusted and seen as the go to guy or girl for advice

2. Do taster sessions in your gym to show a client what you can do. It's the perfect opportunity to highlight your skills and capabilities

3. Join a local business networking group and advertise your services within the group

4. Train the local hairdresser, it may be worth your while training them for free. Hairdressers speak to a lot of clients daily; if you get them the results they've been looking for, they're likely to tell everyone they meet

5. Train owners of a local business, i.e. a trendy new coffee shop that's just opened up in town. Again, you're training people who talk to a lot of customers on a daily basis. That's a lot of people potentially hearing how awesome you are

6. Run a fitness-related charity event in the local area and contact the local newspaper. Have them write an article on what you did for the event and the money you raised and it will inadvertently link to your business and promote you locally. You might also be able to speak about it on the local radio as well, so pitch the segment to them too

7. Network with local businesses and set up initiatives. You could offer a local business 15-minute massages during lunch breaks for 4 employees once a week (that's only 60 minutes of your time). You may even be paid for your efforts if the owner of the company sees this as a well-being initiative for the staff. That gives you an 'in' with 4 new potential clients each week, a chance to build trust

8. Flyer drop to local businesses in your area advertising a taster session for your new bootcamp. Use the flyer as a voucher for free entry, or offer some thing of value, a reason to turn up or contact you

9. Create some form of partnership with a local business or council who are pro moting a popular upcoming event. This is an opportunity to showcase your business to a larger audience with an established organisation or event

10. Have a friends and family referral scheme that encourages people to tell their friends about your business. In return, thank them with a free session or a massage

If you work in a gym or have a gym the strategies above are far quicker, easier and more successful for attracting clients than online marketing. Posting on your Instagram page, blogging on Facebook and filming a YouTube video are less effective forms of advertising for a local business in comparison to getting out there and being seen.

Back to David Lloyd

When I arrived back home to Ipswich and joined the David Lloyd gym, I didn't use a single online marketing tactic to attract new clients. Like most personal trainers, I started with no clients and within 7 weeks I was doing 20 hours of personal training. I chose to hustle and get in front of people.

I worked hard to speak to as many people as possible and build trust with them.

I wanted to be the trainer that gym members could approach and ask for advice.

The actions I carried out in that David Lloyd gym were as follows:

1. I joined a local Business Networking International (BNI) group. It was a great opportunity to attract clients. I paid my membership fee and advertised myself as the group's go-to personal trainer. Within a few weeks I had gained several clients from the group

2. I always hustled on the gym floor during my shifts and tried to speak to as many members as I could. Rather than pitch my skills, I made every effort to help gym members during their workouts and build trust as an expert

3. I wrote a simple 3-page nutrition tips sheet and printed loads of copies out. I then placed them on a wall holder by the gym's noticed board and offered them to members for free. Lots of members took one and this generated interest in the nutrition coaching aspect of my business

4. If I was in the gym training myself, I would offer gym members the opportunity to train alongside me and they loved it. Some signed up for future personal training sessions while others would recommend me to their friends. It generated interest in my business and my name was known around the gym. It was also fun

5. I took pride in cleaning the gym equipment when other trainers didn't. I earned the respect of the members as everyone appreciates a clean and working gym. It's rare to see trainers cleaning gym equipment without looking like a grumpy child being punished!

6. I offered free 10-minute nutrition consultations to every member that I had a gym induction with and gave them a copy of my 3-page nutrition tips sheet. The members really appreciated this gesture; using a little of my time to deliver something of value made me stand out from the other trainers at the gym

7. When I wasn't on a shift, I'd offer a free 10-minute postural analysis or nutrition consultation and I would advertise this ahead of time. I'd give 24 hours' notice and put a sign up in the seating area in the gym that said: 'FREE Nutrition Consultation or postural analysis – 7-8pm Tuesday night'. I'd also attach a time slot sheet for clients to write down their details so I knew who was coming in and when. It was yet another opportunity to provide clients

with a valuable service and allow them the opportunity to build trust with me prior to paying for training sessions

Those were my 7 tactics. It was enough to keep me busy and I built my business up quickly from doing so. None of the above tactics suggest an easy route to getting clients, but let's be honest, none of that was that hard or took loads of extra time, it was just a case of thinking outside the box and putting myself out there a bit.

I could have sat by the gym desk posting selfies or written about my training specialities on Instagram, but it doesn't build rapport as quickly as talking to a prospective client in person.

Attract business for yourself by getting out there and working for it. That doesn't mean cold-calling or pitching your skills; rather, it means sharing your knowledge, using opportunities to help others and when they're ready, letting them come to you.

Then you make an easy sale, they are already in, and it's then just the formalities.

If you don't show someone how AWESOME you are, you give them no reason to train with you. Generate action and show them what you can do for them.

No more hiding behind the walls of the internet with sub-standard online marketing. If you're in a gym, go and talk to the members, create in-house initiatives, create initiatives locally, and convert those people into valued clients.

For those of you who own or work in a smaller gym that doesn't provide you access to 1000s of members, your marketing will require more online content. But I would still like you to refer back to my 10-point list and ensure that you're using some of those tactics to boost your business. Regardless of your working environment, they're still incredibly useful pointers.

Expanding your business knowledge

If you would like to expand your business knowledge in the future, then consider signing up to our The BTN Academy Business Academy. We built this course to equip trainers with a plethora of skills to become competent in all aspects of marketing your personal or fitness brand. And yes, I am selling to you. This book was written to provide you with the guidance to take your personal training to the next level. To advance beyond this book, look to the BTN Business Academy.

But first, you have enough to get on with. This book has enough tips for you to get cracking.

Now it's time to commit to action. Wherever you are right now, you can improve the number of clients you have, even if it's putting them onto a waiting list or optimising your time with semi-private training sessions. Either way, I want you to write down 3 actions you're going to commit to doing as a result of reading this chapter, with the aim of gaining more clients.

I'm going to give you space for 5 actions so that in the future you can build on the first 3:

1. _____

2. _____

3. _____

4. _____

5. _____

Don't take the easy way out with posting online when your clients can be found far easier on the gym floor or in your local community.

Find your client, shake their hand, create a connection, show them your work, spend time and invest in them; I guarantee your business will thrive.

Now stop wasting time and get out there!

CHAPTER 13
THE 6-FIGURE TRAINER

I have absolutely no idea what happened, or why it happened, but over the last 18 months (I sit here writing this in Nov 2016) there's been a sharp rise in the number of internet gurus promising personal trainers the dream of a 6-figure income.

I see a new guru pop up almost every day on Facebook or via email and I can imagine that there's a lot of people out there who have bought into their BS promises. And that's a bit sad, because honestly, can you really make a 6-figure salary in a gym coaching everyday people?

Some can, but the circumstances have to be in your favour. I would say you needed to be:

1. In London, or a big city
2. Very good at your job and at getting results with your clients
3. Have robust systems in place to generate that income
4. Be charging around £75 per hour working a 30-hour week, 11 months of the year, or charging less and working your butt off, so much so that you have no health or quality of life (and that figure doesn't include your gym rent or ANY overheads, so it's more likely to be closer to £90 per hour, 30 hours a week)
5. Have a slick and high quality marketing system
6. Pay very little or next to nothing for your gym space

That's not to say that it can't be done, it can, but expect the stars to align for you and for a lot of external factors to be in your favour.

This chapter isn't an opportunity to hate on people that are successful and to completely dismiss the notion of becoming a 6-figure trainer. Rather, the idea is to bring you back to reality and work on building yourself up to that level, if you so wish.

If I'm a personal trainer in a gym earning £20,000 a year (the industry average is between £16-26,000) then saying or believing that you're going to be a 6-figure trainer is questionable. That's 5 times your current salary and a LOT of optimism.

141

It's not SMART, at least not SMART in the time frame that most want it to happen in.

What is **SMART**?

SMART is a classic method of goal setting. You'll likely have seen it before, especially if you've had a past exposure to goal setting. It's a classic measurement system that stands for:

Specific

Measurable

Attainable

Realistic

Time-bound

Now becoming a 6-figure trainer isn't unattainable, but it probably is if you expect to obtain that within a year. I reckon you could easily go from £20,000 to £40-50,000 a year using the advice I'm giving you in this book, but £100,000 a year? I'm going to be honest, it's highly unlikely.

Dream big, of course. I do and will continue to every day. But do so in a realistic fashion.

You also need to ask yourself what success looks like for you. Why is a 6-figure trainer deemed successful?

Here's an exercise for you. I want you to list 5 things below that describe what success looks like to you, personally:

1. _____

2. _____

3. _____

4. _____

5. _____

How many of your points above are financially orientated, and if so, where did your numbers come from, and why?

For some reason people think becoming a millionaire is a sign of success; it's the golden number. Earn a million and you're immediately happy, all is fulfilled and you can put your feet up, you happy little camper.

Ask someone, go on: "What does financial success look like to you?" I'll bet they'll say :"To be a millionaire".

It's the same with physical success. Many see getting a six pack as the end goal, the pinnacle of getting fit and in shape. But why?

Back to money.

What if you could live an AWESOME life on £40,000 a year as a trainer, or less?

I ask, as once you get over £32,000 ish a year you start to live a VERY comfortable life. You have money for good food, a nice house, nice holidays, clothes, a nice car and most of the things that people strive for in life. It's a good life with little stress when it comes to money and you have the financial backing do the things you've always wanted to do.

Again, I'm not saying don't aim high. Be the best you can be, but if you do the best you possibly can for your clients then you will be successful and create a comfortable lifestyle by default.

Forget about the numbers for now (that comes later) and forget about the big dreams. Let's go back to basics. Go back to the idea of the lock-in: once you've finished this book and reviewed all the necessary chapters, I want you to complete your lock-in.

In the meantime, we'll use an example.

Let's say you're a trainer currently earning £20,000 a year.

Before you get geeky with earning projections and future cash flow, focus on the fundamentals (just like you would get your clients to do). You can't drive a business in terms of numbers without all the foundations in place. You'd be focusing on all the wrong stuff. And at this stage we're not ready for that.

For now, you need to be smart and get the last 12 chapters engrained into your psyche. You need to care for your clients, put systems in place, get confident in your abilities, layer your pricing to entice clients into the business and be the best you can be. Only then can you start to get geeky.

So, let's say you're earning £20,000 per year right now in your gym and are charging £20 per hour working 18 hours per week. Our first port of call would be to boost that client number closer to 25-28.

This puts you in a more comfortable financial position. There's less stress on you and you'll feel generally happier. For now, I don't want you to aim higher and work more than 25-28 contact hours per week. I still want you to have spare time to implement systems and keep working ON your business while also working IN your business.

With the remaining 10-20 working hours that you have free, ensure that you're implementing your systems. Review your customer service strategy and ensure your check-in system works. Confirm that your clients are happy and that you have the time and head space to do all aspects of your job, both IN your business and ON your business.

We don't want to up your clients to 30-35 hours a week just yet as it adds pressure. If your systems are not yet in place and if things are not working 100%, then you don't have the time, head space or focus to fix them or even implement them successfully. Only when your systems and processes become habitual, similar to you client drinking 2 litres of water a day, can we then advance and boost client intake.

We need the foundations to be set so we can build high. Set the foundations first and only then consider taking client numbers from 25-28 up to 35, or thereabouts. At this stage your business will be thriving, you're in a positive financial position and you're challenging all aspects of your business, but they are strong and can be challenged and put under strain.

Once you are at 25-28 hours per week, and you are happy that you have done the work from this book and made your business stronger and robust, then look to boost your client numbers.

Your business is then ready; you've put in the work.

The easy way to put your prices up

35 hours for many trainers is a good place to be: you're busy, you're getting a lot of clients and your business is working with all its systems and strategies in place. At this point in time, you can confidently increase your prices. You're busy and can justify your fee; any new client that comes into your business is now paying £30, or £40 or whatever you feel is fair and a valuable measure of your time. As clients drop off over time, which they will, you can bring new clients in at the new price (hopefully at this point in time you also have a waiting list for your services, now that's a good place to be in!).

So, to recap. You have a full client list, 35 hours a week, anyone new is safe to bring in at the new pricing structure, the demand is there and people can see you are worth what you are charging.

What about your current clients?

At this point you might be thinking "Can I not increase my prices with all my existing clients, I now value my time more and I'd like to put my prices up across the board. I'm in demand?".

Yes, you can, you just need to be tactful.

When increasing your prices with your existing clients, write them all a letter or advise them in-person that the demand for your services is high. Explain that your prices are going up to reflect your ability, level of knowledge now (because you have been doing lots of extra training and CPD) and the value of the service you offer to them has improved.

Then give them a date that your prices will go up from and give them fair warning.

You can't do this overnight, and you should honour any existing contracts or up-front payments you have, such as people that have bought a block of 10 sessions at a set price.

Now be warned, some of your clients WILL leave, and that is ok. If you're putting your prices up from £20 to £30, for example, and 35% of your clients leave, you're still earning the same money but are working less hours.

Win win.

In saying that, when any of your clients do leave your services, go back to your foundations and reflect honestly on your performance. Were you getting good results with them? Were they happy and were you a good trainer to them? Or was it purely financially related and they weren't willing to pay more?

£20 to £30 might be a big jump for your clients, and also for you. If this is the case go slower and increase to a price that you feel comfortable with, perhaps going from £20 to £25 initially, and then look to perform another jump 6 months later.

Whatever approach you decide on, be assured of your abilities and respect your time; be confident in the value of your service and never feel scared to charge what you're worth. If you are AWESOME at your job, people will always pay for your time. Please don't under value yourself.

Should you gain some free time during your price increase due to the loss of a few clients, use this time wisely to work on a new phase of optimising your business. You could start to implement some semi-private training sessions during your price increase, or even better plan this into your price increase offering.

Let's say you were charging £20 an hour and increasing to £30 an hour for your 1-2-1 sessions. You can now offer semi-private training session as £20 per hour where you will be training small groups of 3 or 4 people. This then gives you the chance to boost your income for the same amount of time and your clients can still train with you without it costing them more money.

Without focusing too much on the money at this point in time, good things have happened. You've improved your client numbers by implementing more hustle on the gym floor. By using a few tactics, you're improving the delivery of your customer service system and now that you're comfortable with your foundations, you can make a second boost for more clients to increase your working hours. Once this boost has occurred, you can safely put your prices up using a new pricing structure and introduce newer options of semi-private training, group training and class packages.

No matter what stage you're at, your business needs to be kept simple. It needs to be adaptable to your gym environment and the resources you have at your disposal.

At this point a personal trainer might get greedy and I don't think this is a problem short-term. You're wanting push for more clients and a greater income, but be careful of the long-term consequences of greed.

Why?

Imagine the scenario. You get a taste of having a bigger and better level of income so you push for 40 clients a week and put your prices up again. Your client numbers drop to 30 and you then push for more clients again. You might then repeat this process several times throughout the year until you get to 40 hours or more on the gym floor and stay there.

What quality of life do you expect to have working those hours? Will you have good work-life balance?

As a personal trainer, 40 hours on the gym floor isn't 40 hours of work; when you factor in emails to send, programs to design, texts to answer, calls, and all the other admin tasks that come with a thriving business. It's more like 50, 55 or maybe even 60 hours a week. It's vitally important that you take into account the total hours working in your business, not just your paid hours.

This is where you need to get in tune with the numbers of your business and the lifestyle that you want to create. Sure, work all the hours of the day and make as much money as possible, but are those long hours really what you want long-term?

Is it healthy?

You might do it short-term to save up for a house, a new car or something you really want in life, but I don't believe this is healthy or sustainable for years on end.

You'll burnout, lose your love for personal training, and this will cause a decline in the service you give to your clients. We need to maintain quality of service, so work life balance is key.

So, I'll raise a very important question, how much money do you actually need to live the life you want to lead?

Your outgoings per month might look like this:

Mortgage / rent:	£600.00
Bills:	£100.00
Food:	£300.00
Car:	£100.00
Fuel:	£150.00
Sundries:	£250.00
Spending:	£250.00
Total:	£1750.00

Hypothetically, that's how much you spend each month on the necessary expenses that come with living your month to month life. Let's say on top of that you want to save £500 a month for a new house and have £250 a month saved for holidays and other stuff. That's an extra £750 a month you need.

In order to live the life that you want and to save, live, explore and be happy, you need £2500 per month, which is £30,000 a year.

I'd actually aim for £3360.00 ish per month. That's £300 extra per month to account for holidays and £560.00 extra for your tax (tax calculated at 20%). We always need holidays as you don't get paid for holiday, and you MUST pay your tax, so always factor that in.

See, I told you things get comfortable and life is good at around £32,000 a year. The above example acts as a guideline so by all means adapt this information to your own environment, conditions, rules, dreams and wants. But you can see what I'm doing here. I'm planning your finances strategically so you know how much you actually need to earn to live the life you want. This is so you don't end up working 60 hours a week spinning your wheels just trying to earn as much as humanly possible with the available hours in the day, which most coaches do. Instead you optimise your business so you are working 25-30 hours per week (client contact time) earning what you need to earn with happy clients, an optimised business and good work life balance.

You can then factor those figures into your business in a more strategic fashion. To earn £32,000 a year means working 30 hours a week at £22 an hour on average. Again, those prices and hours will vary depending on what you deem to be an optimal fit for your lifestyle.

Not enough personal trainers lock-in and create a plan like this. When I was a trainer in the early days, I lived hand to mouth, cash-in-hand payment to cash-in-hand payment. I was sloppy with my money and only worked when my clients needed me. I spent whatever money I had and sacrificed my lifestyle to suit my earnings. There was no consistency and I didn't have any control over my business.

So plan.

What do you want to earn?

How many hours a week is that?

How much do you need to charge per hour?

And when you get there, look to optimise it again based on demand for your time and your ability to maximise your income, thus eventually boosting your income methodically, in a realistic and achievable way.

Call the shots early doors

In the early days of building up your business, you're going to work a lot and you will often have to work at random times to appease your clients. But when you start to see success, you're in a position to call the shots and bring some control back into your business and to your lifestyle.

If you get to a point where you're working 25-30 hours a week with time to strategise and optimise your business, and can afford to lose a few clients for a greater work-life balance, do it.

If you're currently working all over the place for your clients (early mornings, late nights, random afternoon sessions) and you want to tighten your schedule, do it.

If you want to work like this:

Mondays - 6-10am and 4-8pm

Tuesday - 6-10am and 4-8pm

Wednesday - 7-10am

Thursday - 6-11am and 4-8pm

Friday - 6am-2pm

Then do it: call the shots.

You have to enforce some boundaries on your time, I do it. I have to. Let's say you want to schedule an hour mentoring time with me, and you're going to pay for an hour of my time. I'm in the position of power to arrange that call to a time that works around me and my business. If I was starting off in my career and building up my name, then for a time I would let you, the client, call the shots and I'd accommodate your availability. But this isn't the case now. I dictate my own working hours and you have to fit into that time. If I didn't do that I'd be unable to maintain my quality of life and my work-life balance.

I personally work:

Monday: 7am-9pm with a 2 hour break for training and 2x 20 minute dog walks

Tuesday: 7am-5pm with 2x 20 minute dog walks. I then have rugby training in the evening

Wednesday: 7am-2pm. A shorter day to allow for date night

Thursday: 7am-5pm with 2x 20 minute dog walks. Like Tuesday, I have rugby training in the evening

Friday: Variable, but often 7am-1pm

I sometimes work in the early mornings of the weekend on projects or writing as I have the clarity and space to think during that time. I may also be working away at the weekend. If this is the case, I take more time off during the week to balance out my work time if the schedule isn't too packed with essential stuff to do.

So, I have my boundaries, if you want me at 4pm on a Wednesday you can't have me. This also applies to 6pm on a Tuesday. You get the picture. I have to have boundaries to cater for my wants, my work-life balance and my lifestyle. But I still work hard and I still work a fair bit. I also mainly work from home so I don't have much commuting time: this allows me to optimise my working environment.

I still work approximately 40-50 hours per week, sometimes far more, because I love my job and I'm on a mission, but I could easily choose to work less and do less. I choose to do what I do and it works for me. It gives me enough time to work and earn, but also to create new projects and develop the business: splitting my time between working IN the business and ON the business.

So be objective, see the path and the needs of your business. Have your lock-in, work out your plan and outline your path.

I have given you a very clear and simple framework to follow here, and it will work.

Have faith in yourself and your abilities.

Take things slowly; dream big, but be realistic.

Master your craft and business as a personal trainer.

Build things up in phases and make the next move with your business structure and costs when you move into a positon of greater power.

By all means be a 6-figure personal trainer, but don't consider a higher financial sum to be a sign of success. Success can come at a much lower price and you have the power to define your success, not some guru.

CHAPTER 14
WHAT YOUR CLIENTS SAY ABOUT YOU

This chapter is an ode to your clients.

If I'm going to write a book about being better at your job, sorry, AWESOME at your job, don't you think I should find out what your clients dislike about you?

Sometimes we need to be told what's wrong and often change only happens when it's spelled out to us and shoved in our faces. This is what this chapter is about. So far, this book has been written in a way that highlights key fundamentals for developing you as a better personal trainer. The next logical step is to ask your clients to highlight problems in our industry and with what we do as coaches.

If your client is picking up on the following behaviours, then you MUST change them; you would be a complete idiot not too. Remember, everything you do is for the client, the person paying for your time. It's not for you, your gains, or your finances; it's for your client.

If you don't act in the interests of your client, and you're not genuinely passionate about your job and what you do, then cease being a personal trainer. I'm only saying this because everyone should follow their passion in life. I'm following my passion now by being a writer, speaker and educator to others. The day I stop wanting to wake up every day and do it all over again is the day I need to do something else.

When I talk, you can see my passion and it makes the words that I say that much more meaningful. If I wasn't passionate, if I didn't speak with conviction and I didn't have this energy about what I did, then I wouldn't inspire you half as much as I do. People can see and feel passion. It's infectious.

Apathy taints the industry I love and have worked so hard to add value to, and passion is an essential character trait of being the best trainer that you can be.

Never do a job you dislike; stand up, be honest with yourself, and change career paths. Don't feel bad about your decision, it's just the truth, and we deserve to live out our truth.

In this chapter I have also listed some comments from fellow personal trainers as they're genuine observations that I also agree with. You'll find those comments after the section from clients.

But firstly, how did I conduct this research?

On 21st November 2016 on my 'Ben Coomber' Facebook page I asked the following question:

"I'm book writing today and I'm interested...

What do you see Personal Trainers and Coaches doing online and offline, that you hate?

It could be anything, I'm all ears...

You will be shaping a VERY important chapter in the book and will get a mention!"

Off the back of this post I got 168 comments from people who wanted to give their opinions; I have directly quoted some of the comments below and thus credited all the people who took the time to respond.

Which leads me to say a massive THANK YOU to all the people that support my work. The likes you give on my posts, the shares, the comments, the shout-outs, the selfies we have at events, the people that attend my talks, the positive comments we get about The BTN Academy, the reviews and the people that write into the podcast. Thank you all; your support is invaluable and I look forward to serving you even more over the coming years.

The research

How do we know my research is credible?

At the time of making this post my Facebook page had around 64,000 followers, so we can trust that we have a broad account of people's opinions. Many of these comments were also supported with a lot of likes, often 50-100 people backing up the initial comment. These comments are genuine, from real people with an opinion to share.

So, without further delay, this is what your clients dislike about you with my input following each comment.

Comments from your clients

Alex Lawrence: *I see a lot of personal trainers playing on their phones and not watching a client's form or technique. Also, not engaging in conversation with the client irritates me, sometimes clients can't talk when they are working hard, but on rest/recovery period you can engage in a conversation, strike up a long-lasting friendship with your clients. Talk about why they are doing that and give little pointers.*

Hallelujah! I'm glad someone brought up mobile phone usage early in the discussion. I personally find it despicable when a trainer is flicking through Instagram when a client is resting. That client is paying for your time, not for you to sit on Instagram looking at food pictures and celebrity selfies. Unless it's on flight mode and your phone is being used to track the client's progress, put the phone away. It's unacceptable to ignore your client just because they're on a rest period; it's also VERY unprofessional. If you are using your phone to track a work-out during a session and don't want to appear uncaring, consider using an iPad or tablet instead to avoid any misconceptions from onlookers.

Pete Goldsmith: *Multi-layer marketing: He****ife, J***e P**s, and all those types of companies really grind my gears - especially when the person doing the selling either has a) zero knowledge, or b) enough knowledge to know better!*

I've been very vocal in the past with companies of this nature; if you take a look at my YouTube account, I've shared my thoughts on MLM-based products and I've also written plenty of blogs on this topic. My issue with MLM lies in the selling practices of the products, the lack of knowledge and the claims from certain products which are both unethical and completely false. As I mentioned in a previous chapter, choose to work with supplement companies, and companies in general, that have similar values to your business and seek to earn an affiliate or trade account fee from your support. You may earn less than the MLM junk, but at least you'll have your ethics intact and will sleep easy at night.

Val Allen: *Bad mouthing other coaches/personal trainers who maybe do things differently. Slagging off Zumba/Yoga/Pilates etc. It's disrespectful to the instructors and the people who do them. We all do different types of exercise for different reasons and in my opinion, anything is better than nothing. It all depends on what you enjoy and what your goals are.*

BOOM! I love this. There are many ways to skin a cat; the key aims of our industry are to get people moving, get them healthy and get them happy. If Zumba gets somebody fit and makes them happy, then what's the issue? You might have your way that works for you and your body, but that won't work for everyone. For example, I love the gym but my girlfriend doesn't. She hates it and hasn't been for years. Instead, she plays her sport 5 times a week and plays at national level. Should she be forced to use a gym? Always give a solution that's fun and appropriate for an individual's goals and can be maintained over the long-term.

Anthony Mc Nally: *I don't like seeing personal trainers do the following:*

- *Providing nutritional plans that are not only dangerous but that they have no qualifications to back them up*
- *Doing hands-on massage techniques when they don't have a massage qualification*
- *Focusing so much on aesthetics that their clients think this is what training is about (what about feeling good, sleeping better, energy, movement, quality of life?)*

That's the top 3 for now, I could list more... ;)

It goes without saying that you need to be qualified to teach and do what you do as a trainer, otherwise, if you're not insured to practice then you're liable for malpractice if something goes wrong. Cover your back and don't risk practicing outside of your remit. As for nutritional plans, always make them safe, enjoyable, sustainable and life enhancing. And keep them simple.

Michele Pollard: *I was massively overweight (now just overweight) and had some sessions with a personal trainer who made me feel I was worthless and was wasting his time, who also scoffed at me when I asked if I should use a personal trainer. I was close to giving up the gym as I was totally demotivated by him. I then met a fantastic personal trainer who has provided me with support, encouragement and empathy - he also doesn't take any bullshit or excuses and since training with him he has helped me lose 5 stone. I still have a long way to go but am certain I will get there!*

I fully believe the key to a great PT is actually caring about your clients and their goals and being able to tailor your approach to help them get there. My PT has been so encouraging that I've actually signed up to your BTN foundation course next year so I can improve my own knowledge!

Proof is in the pudding right there! A personal trainer can either inspire and encourage, or put people off for life. I've been guilty of neglecting my clients' needs in the past and I've explained my concerns over that. Respect the power you have as a trainer and use that power with responsibility.

Michelle Halcrow: *I went to a weights class – when I walked in it was full of men setting up so I did the same and the trainer said to me: "This isn't fat blast". Whoa!!! Luckily I'm thick skinned as well as thick waisted (yes I'm female and I'm working on my waist which is why I was there in the 1st place!) and so I said: "I know," and stayed for the class. I think if he'd have said: "Welcome, nice to see more women doing weights," I might have been back – meathead!*

Again, you have the power to inspire others, use that power wisely!

Liam Duncan: *My biggest thing I hate about personal training is the so called personal trainers who have lifted weights a few times or have done a bodybuilding competition and then think that it qualifies them to train other people!*

Yes, they have worked hard to get their body but their methods might not be applicable to others, and without the knowledge and training you're playing a very dangerous game.

I dislike this too. Just because you can get into shape doesn't give you the automatic ability to train others. It can give you a better grounding of the gym environment as you know what it takes in terms of work ethic, training intensity, periodisation and diet. But as this book has highlighted, personal training is MUCH more than just applying diet and training theory to any willing and paying client.

Maciej Matuszak: *My pet peeve is not really what my personal trainer is doing, more what other people do while I'm training with him. I like him as a trainer, he's very friendly and he seems to know everyone in the gym. So what happens is that often during my session people will be coming up to him to chat. Now, I don't mind when people just come up to say "hello", but I do mind when it turns into full conversation during which I end up doing the whole set without my trainer even looking at me and then I still have to wait for them to finish talking.*

Or like today, when in the middle of my workout a guy comes up and asks my PT to demonstrate an exercise for him. I'm paying good money for a 1 on 1 session to have the attention on me. And like I said, it's not necessarily what my trainer does, just other people. In the previous gym I went to, trainers would often wear shirts that said 'I'm training a client'.

In this situation, the trainer is responsible. By all means be polite and say hello to other members, but it is then your responsibility to say: "I'll talk to you later, I'm training a client right now, I'm free at X time or drop me a text later". Your client's session should be focused on the client, not anyone else. Be polite to the person, and then focus back on the client.

Giorgio Esposito: *I HATE when personal trainers don't carry any form of plan around with them for their clients. So many times, I see personal trainers train clients without any form of tracking or planning. They just walk around to a different machine with no structure. How do they remember what weight their clients lifted? What equipment was used? Surely they can't see progress if there's no use of tracking? Not even a pen and paper at least.*

If you want to chart a client's progress, then a plan is crucial. A plan may not be necessary if the session is focused on general movement and mixing up training ideas. But as soon as the client advances a little, you should have a plan for their progression with you.

Lindsey Shimmy Abbott: *I get so infuriated by personal trainers or class instructors who are more focused on themselves than the participant. Ultimately, we 'should' try to be a role model, but keep it real. No fads, no egos.*

You may think others don't notice your ego, but they do. Or perhaps certain trainers are so wrapped up in themselves that they genuinely don't notice. It's something I see all the time in the bodybuilding world and it's sad; stop flexing your muscles in the mirror as you go to pick up a weight. Get over yourself, get rid of your insecurities and focus on your client.

Steve Geoghegan: *I see a lot of personal trainers only approach females and don't look further afield for client's because they assume we are all on track and know what we are doing. I've been training 14 years on and off and a personal trainer approached me for the first time last week. In all those years, I must have given off a bad vibe, who knows. The very fact he engaged in conversion with me he got to understand that I'm not where I want to be and actually the guy or girl who works hard is the one that will be good for business long term for them. Conversation goes a long way.*

As I've mentioned in the earlier chapters, never pass judgement. Everyone is a potential client and you never know when someone needs help with their training or diet.

Kirsty Taylor: *I don't see my personal trainer doing anything I don't like because he is a f***ing legend! I'm a lucky girl. But I frequently watch trainers in a high street gym ignore poor form while giving positive feedback, I know everyone needs encouragement but in the right places, it's no help to anyone to tell someone they have nailed it when they are planking with a dropping spine or blatantly flailing all over the place trying to do an exercise.*

Teaching good form is essential for your client's safety and I hope that is what they are teaching you on the level 3 personal training courses. Always pay attention to your client's movement patterns.

Katy Shenton: *Moaning about 'fat people' it's really annoying especially since a lot of people go to them for fat loss! Each client is different; some people respond better to negative feedback some respond better to positive. Learn which suits each client.*

Word.

Richard Ling: *Doing a cheeky workout behind the clients back while they are doing there set this not paying attention, saw a personal trainer yesterday behind a client who was doing a seated row and just did pull ups without watching.*

No. Just no.

Chris Powles: *Asking you to get off a machine you got to first so the personal trainer can continue a program with the client. I don't like being told I can't do my last set because your client needs it so specifically on time when there's nothing around the machine saying so.*

Respect other members in the gym, they pay to be there too. Be friendly and ask to use the equipment as you would in your own training session. You never know, you may impress that member with your training demeanour and they may consider you to train them one day. Always be polite.

Sam Utting: *I hate to see personal trainers who are unable to demonstrate what they are trying to get their clients to do with proper form. I don't think a personal trainer should be able to do everything, but I think they should be honest and teach what they can teach clients well and above all safely.*

If you can't demonstrate an exercise properly, how do you expect the client learn it properly?

Andy Hillocks: *Not respecting the facility that they work at. For example, leaving weights on bars, not putting dumbbells back.*

Respect and take pride in your place of work. It's a good habit to get into and it's part of your duties as a trainer within a gym.

Jen Doherty: *When personal trainers post unnatural before and after shots of themselves and clients. We all know a bit of fake tan can bring out the best. But a mirror selfie as a before then a professional shot done with fake tan, different pose etc, it actually gives you false hope if you're an everyday joe looking to lose* *weight and tone as it's not a true picture of progression!*

I think this comes down to being real and honest about what you do and what you are promoting. Does your client want to tan and do a photoshoot? It's just a thought, I know I wouldn't.

Daniel John: *Personal Trainers wearing their little brothers t shirt. Trying to impress rather than coach. Lack of professionalism and low standards.*

It's painful to watch. If only you could see yourself...oh wait, the gym is full of mirrors and you know it!

Dave Potter: *Seeing, especially on Snapchat, trainers are taking videos of clients and posting on their story, but the client's technique is away off!*

If you're going to post something online to promote what you do, make sure it's correct and legitimate, otherwise you're just going to look foolish and set yourself up for scrutiny.

Jason Hynes: *Living in a gym bubble. They can sometimes miss the fact that not everyone works in a gym. They'll repeat the notion that "everyone has an hour to work out, just an hour". What they don't realise is that an hour to workout is 15 mins getting ready, half hour driving to the gym, a 15 mins-half hour showering/changing afterwards and a half hour driving home. Makes "just an hour" over 2 hours, maybe close to 3 hours.*

I love this, it's so true. Remember, clients live in their world and have problems, that are their own.

Serge Dalhuysen: *Trainers of athletes who do not have a clue what it's like training obese, depressed, drinking, smoking, injured, not motivated, untalented, sleep deprived, stressed out, overworked, people. Real people with careers, families and 60-hour workweeks.*

Trainers only impress themselves when they train an athlete. In reality, athletes are the easiest people to train, trust me, I've trained plenty. They're motivated, driven, have great genetics and are ready to change; you just need to give them the plan. The everyday client struggles with a multitude of issues and that's where your true skill as a trainer comes into practice.

Ross Yeoman:

1) *The "go hard or go home" mentality*

2) *Not educating clients and just "instructing"*

3) *Ranting because they struggle to make money and aren't willing to change what they do*

4) *Not understanding that clients have a social life too*

5) *Using pyramid schemes and hijacking Instagram to sell stuff*

6) *Believing that they are "holier than thou" when in fact we are all in it to improve our lives*

Succinct and direct, I like it.

Comments from other personal trainers

Jamie Adams: *Trainers that try to get 'first timer 30-year old Jenny' doing the new workout craze when she doesn't even know how to squat #foundationsfirst*

I will refer to the KISS your clients chapter here. Simplify everything for your client and don't advance them any further than they need to. Build from the foundations and focus on getting them moving, losing weight and feeling fit.

Will Humphreys: *No programming, I often see personal trainers doing the same session, with same resistance in the same order for weeks on end. They focus on the session and not the program.*

And, a lack of coaching, just putting people on a machine and telling them to do a movement they've probably never done before without adequate demonstration and explanation of what it's doing and why it relates to them and their goal.

If this is the case then you need to go back to your personal training course books and re-visit periodsation; it's one of the basic ways the body adapts and responds. And if you're not demonstrating an exercise adequately for a client, then I would say you lack passion for your job. Find that passion or move on.

Graham Grice: *The phone issue but in reverse...not telling the client to "put that bloody phone away or you can have your money back and hire somebody else". One of my stipulations if I was training someone would be no phones while training.*

Good reversal on the phone rule! The client is there to focus so unless something is pressing or urgent while they're training (issues at work, kids etc), be firm and have them commit to their session.

Edward Ley: *Criticising what other personal trainers are doing publicly without any idea of what that trainer is trying to achieve with their client.*

Don't get me wrong, I've done it, but over time I've realised that there are many ways to train someone and to onlookers it can appear that you are neglecting something, when in reality you merely have a different perspective.

In this case I think a bit more humility is needed.

Physiotherapy, Chiropractic, Osteopathy: These professions are less quick to criticise people and techniques and spend more time trying to understand and add to their knowledge base, or see the other person's perspective.

I think this approach would be one that might move personal training from amateur to professional. But I'm willing to accept that I could be wrong...

There are many ways to skin a cat. If you don't understand why or how in any given situation, you are just passing unreasonable judgement on someone and their methods.

Kate Harper: *I have a large gym in Tenerife, we have everything from fat loss clients to competing bodybuilders and fighters. We also have trainers from all* over Europe, all with different ideas and methods. The two things that stand out for me are making clients do strange exercises (usually involving balancing!) so that they think they have achieved something but in reality, they cannot remember how to do it again, have no idea why they did it, and it took so long to set up each time it was probably as waste of time. This goes on to my next pet peeve... trainers who train themselves properly, but give their clients programs that are truly bizarre – maybe so that the client will always need the trainer, as it has been so over-complicated.

For us, the best trainers educate clients. Give them a solid program and explain why you do what you do, why you do X sets and X reps, why you sometimes do a light / really heavy week. Explain what progress you want to see, measure it along the way. Tell them when and why you change things and why you do what you do. Work together.

Some great input from a gym owner and seasoned trainer.

Ben Gray: *Spending time trying to impress other personal trainers and 'gurus' rather than focusing on their own message and how they can help clients/ potential clients get the results they want.*

Word. Stop trying to impress others. It's all too common in an industry that is often full of people trying to prove a point. Look at the bigger picture: it's not about you, it's about the client.

Natalie Morley: *Personal trainers taking on any client with zero responsibility/ respect for their needs and goals, but purely for the money. i.e. if you are not qualified to do full rehab program in conjunction with other specialists for a client who has had back surgery or an injury, DON'T TAKE ON THE CLIENT. Personal trainers taking on any business whether they're qualified or not, just for the money.*

Big no-no. Know your remit of practice and work with other professionals to provide the best possible service for the client.

Phil Paterson: *Probably one of the biggest problems I have with many trainers is a lack of willingness to progress their knowledge and professional status. So* many are happy to get their 4-week qualification and train with that base knowledge for years and years with blinkers on to the evolution of the industry around them which changes all the time and we are now in a world where you can learn a ton and be really good at your job (it's one reason I think the BTN academy is such a good tool for personal trainers).

When you work in a group with lots of variety you naturally pick things up. But this can only last so long, since a small group within one gym will see little influence from the outside and then you see them training their clients the same way they did 4 years ago. No development or progression.

I see trainers who've been in the industry for years that if I start talking to them about the progression of movement patterns into sling systems, it looks like their head will explode. Yeah, squats are great, but unless your client jumps to work there's got to be some progression in there. #rant

Education is key. You can't finish your level 3 personal training course and stop there. Take the time to settle into that knowledge, work on your skills and brush up on your business. Only then should you advance yourself and commit to a strength and conditioning course, movement course, the BTN Academy, an annual conference, conventions or exposure yourself to NLP and mindset work. It's the only way you will become an AWESOME personal trainer (as well as applying the skills from this book).

I'll add in a final comment: I have a gripe with trainers who use performance enhancing drugs and claim to be natural. I don't like liars, no one does. This industry needs more honesty, especially for the client who looks up to you for guidance. You're leading that client into a pit of false hope. It's spineless, unethical and totally disrespectful. Be honest, people respect it, and people need to be inspired by what's natural, as that line between natural and unnatural results is now very confusing for everyone training towards a fitness goal.

Wrap up

This is a chapter we can't ignore, and I took a direct approach to this for a reason. In our businesses as personal trainers, we need to be:

1 Self-aware

2 Aware of what our clients want and their perceptions of our training skills

Only then can we truly be great at what we do.

OUTRODUCTION

That's the opposite to an introduction, right? Who knows. I'm making the rules here; it's my book so let's call it an Outroduction!

Rebel I know.

I'm hoping that there are many aspects of this book that you can relate to. I've been direct, I've been empathetic and at times I've been downright harsh. There are some things our industry needs to hear and we shouldn't dance around those subjects. Life's too short for BS.

The personal training industry needs to do better. Speak to any personal training client and you get a mixed bag of opinions: some good, some bad, some great. But rarely awesome.

I want all personal trainers to be AWESOME.

Why?

Because it plays into my mission for the industry. I want to make as many people as AWESOME as humanly possible. If I make you more awesome at your job, you go on to help more people. It produces a massive domino effect of more people losing weight, getting healthy, getting fit, becoming pain free, and generally living a better, more fulfilling, more AWESOME life.

We're here to make a difference, aren't we?

This book aims to question your role in life: can you do a better job?

Do you want to be better?

I hope you do, we owe it to ourselves to be the best we can be.

I want you to be AWESOME.

I want all the clients you help to be AWESOME.

And I want us to collectively combat the bigger issues: obesity, disease, unhappiness, pain, poor movement, lack of fitness, however you want to shape it, the world and the people in it could be in a much better place. And bettering our industry will help in that battle.

Choose to be AWESOME and you stand an infinitely better chance of infecting others with that AWESOMENESS.

Stop the bitching online.

Stop arguing about stuff that just doesn't matter.

Treat everyone as an individual.

Look after your clients, care for them.

Be empathetic.

Put your phone away and focus on the client.

Work to get your clients out of pain and towards a positive emotional state.

Treat your client like a person, and appreciate their real life issues.

Stop acting with ego and instead act with passion and humility.

Keep things simple for your client, help them to live a fitter life.

Be there for them, support them, don't judge.

Quit flexing in the mirror and taking selfies with your top off. Get a handle on your insecurities and do things for the right reasons at the right time.

Quit selling crappy shake diets and diet products because you lack nutrition expertise.

Rant over.

It's time for us all to step up. We have great power as fitness professionals; we hold the nation's health in our hands. Don't abuse that power, treat it with respect and always do the right thing.

Here's to being an AWESOME personal trainer.

Good luck, and see you in...

How to be an AWESOME-ER Personal Trainer (part 2)

How can I help you after today?

Search for 'How to be an Awesome Personal Trainer – Secret FB Group' on Facebook, join the group, and get on-going help from me and the community, and access to a secret video seminar that will help you even more.

Ben Coomber Radio – My #1 rated health and fitness podcast, available on iTunes and other podcasting apps and media players

All over social media – Facebook, Instagram, YouTube, my website - if all this social media stuff is still around by the time you read this book!

My website: www.bencoomber.com

The BTN Academy – For when you decide to take your nutrition education to the next level, we're here for you: btn.academy

Awesome Supplements – If you want to use an ethical supplement brand that's research proven and honest in everything that it does, while simplifying and innovating in the world of supplementation: www.awesomesupplements.co.uk

Other books I have written to date available at www.bencoomber.com:

The Nutrition Blueprint
The Sports Nutrition Blueprint
A Beginners Guide To Lifting Weights
An Intermediates Guide To Lifting Weights
Nutrition For Kids

As well as many other short books, e-books and other beneficial musings online, have a hunt around and I promise you'll find lots of good stuff!

After that, see you in part 2 of this book series...